Secrets of a Former Fat Girl

Secrets of a Former Fat Girl

How to Lose Two, Four (or More!) Dress
Sizes—and Find Yourself Along the Way

Lisa Delaney

HUDSON
STREET
PRESS

HUDSON STREET PRESS
Published by Penguin Group
Penguin Group (USA) Inc., 375 Hudson Street, New York, New York 10014, U.S.A.
Penguin Group (Canada), 90 Eglinton Avenue East, Suite 700, Toronto, Ontario,
Canada M4P 2Y3 (a division of Pearson Penguin Canada Inc.)
Penguin Books Ltd, 80 Strand, London WC2R 0RL, England
Penguin Ireland, 25 St. Stephen's Green, Dublin 2, Ireland
(a division of Penguin Books Ltd.)
Penguin Group (Australia), 250 Camberwell Road, Camberwell, Victoria 3124, Australia
(a division of Pearson Australia Group Pty. Ltd.)
Penguin Books India Pvt. Ltd., 11 Community Centre, Panchsheel Park,
New Delhi – 110 017, India
Penguin Books (NZ), cnr Airborne and Rosedale Roads, Albany, Auckland 1310,
New Zealand (a division of Pearson New Zealand Ltd.)
Penguin Books (South Africa) (Pty.) Ltd., 24 Sturdee Avenue, Rosebank,
Johannesburg 2196, South Africa

Penguin Books Ltd., Registered Offices: 80 Strand, London WC2R 0RL, England

First published by Hudson Street Press, a member of Penguin Group (USA) Inc.

First Printing, April 2007
3   5   7   9   10   8   6   4

Copyright © Lisa Delaney, 2007
All rights reserved

REGISTERED TRADEMARK—MARCA REGISTRADA
HUDSON
STREET
PRESS

LIBRARY OF CONGRESS CATALOGING-IN-PUBLICATION DATA

Delaney, Lisa.
Secrets of a former fat girl : how to lose, two four (or more!) dress sizes, and find
yourself along the way / Lisa Delaney.
p. cm.
ISBN 978-1-59463-033-0 (alk. paper)   1. Weight loss—Anecdotes.   2. Weight
loss—Humor.   3. Delaney, Lisa.   I. Title
RM222.2.D456 2007
613.2'5—dc22
                                        2006026589

Printed in the United States of America
Set in Bembo
Designed by Spring Hoteling

For Rick and Johnny
and Mom and Dad

Contents

Introduction

You don't know me, but you probably hate me.

I'm the girl in the size 2 jeans with the ten marathon medals hanging on the wall, the girl who cracks the joke that gets the whole room laughing, the girl who never goes without her daily chocolate fix and looks as if she doesn't know the meaning of the word *diet*.

You don't know me, but I know you. I know you because I *was* you. Because, despite my tight butt and bikini-worthy abs, I am a Former Fat Girl.

I was a chubby kid who became an even chubbier teen and then just a plain fat adult. I can still feel the stings of my childhood. There was the time in third grade when Mary Ann—the one girl I thought was bigger than me—said that according to her mom *I* was the fattest in the class. There was the shame I felt at the discovery of the goodies I stashed under my bed, in my closet, in my underwear drawer to feed my insatiable sweet tooth. There were the humiliating battles over clothes shopping with my mom, who gently tried to steer me away from the hip-huggers and peasant tops I desperately wanted to wear but that, with my bloated belly, made me look as if I was about to be shipped off to a home for unwed mothers.

I would sneak sweets whenever and wherever I could. On weekdays after school, as my brothers and I gathered around the TV for some mind-numbing cartoons, I'd announce that I was heading to the pantry for "a couple of saltines," or "a handful of Cheez Nips." Casually lingering, I would rummage around for the Chips Ahoy or Oreos or whatever sweet I could lay my hands on, and slip as many into my pocket or up my sleeve as I could without creating an obvious bulge (as if anyone would have noticed another one). Then I'd steal away to my room or even the bathroom where I could lock out my nosy brothers and wolf down my stash. I was like a bulimic who just never got around to the purging part.

My brothers still bring up one particularly painful incident. I was in junior high, which is painful enough in itself, and even more so for us Fat Girls, and we were vacationing at a beach house. A rental with shabby mismatched furniture obviously discarded from the owner's landlocked home, it was the perfect place for our family of seven, including four teenagers and a toddler who couldn't help but rough up the place. Dessert was a layer cake with chocolate butter cream, and not the kind from the can, mind you. (I don't think they even made the stuff back then.) I had finished my piece, scraping the plate to get every last smudge of the gooey frosting. Just out of reach in the center of the table was the remaining quarter of the cake.

My mom and my brothers had started clearing the table, and Dad had risen to go out for a smoke. I saw my chance: I rose, deftly swiped my finger through the frosting at the base of the cake, and was bringing it to my lips when one of my brothers saw me and yelled, *"Lisa's picking at the cake!"* Startled and completely shamed, I plopped back down in my chair, and the damn thing broke. I mean *broke*. The legs gave way, the seat blew out, and I landed in a lump on the floor. What happened was devastating enough, but then I had to endure the laughter that such a pratfall like that just begged for. I wanted to scuttle away into a hole like one of the sand crabs we had spent the day stalking.

And that's kind of what I did. Even before the Summer of the Broken Chair, I had gotten good at hiding. I hid physically, literally, holing up in my room, listening to James Taylor and Elton John albums and writing bad poetry. During high school and college, when I actually had some friends and something of a social life, my hiding was more emotional. Anytime I had something to say, I either kept my mouth shut or muttered the quip under my breath on the off chance that someone around me might hear. I couldn't step out there and risk a joke falling flat, like I fell flat with that flimsy dining room chair. I couldn't even let loose enough to laugh out loud, and when I smiled, I covered my mouth with my hand.

And all the while, on some level, I was hiding under the layers of fat that I allowed to engulf me like a cocoon of comfort.

I might have covered my mouth to stifle a smile, but nothing could stand between it and a morsel of food. Oh, I tried. I swore off chocolate and swore at the scale at every weigh-in when that damn needle refused to budge—or, worse, when it inched up. I tried to exercise and was fairly successful for a brief time in high school when I would run under cover of darkness with my little mutt, Daisy. I even ventured onto a tennis court every once in a while with a couple of friends. (Those were the Chris Evert/Billy Jean King years of tennis when there was this kind of fairy-tale fascination with the sport. But I believe my somewhat pitiful efforts were due to the dreams I had of marrying John McEnroe.)

Gluttony won over love and exercise when I got to college—and I don't use the word *gluttony* lightly. One of our regular haunts was a place that served $5 pitchers of vile but extremely potent Long Island Iced Tea on Wednesday nights. The real draw for me, though, were the nachos; a platter of chips piled a foot high, topped with neon orange cheese sauce and studded with jalapeños. We'd work away at the pile until the sauce was gone, and then we'd ask the server to top it off with more. They always did—at least once, maybe more.

The all-time best example of pigging out, though, came during my freshman year. I was friends with a group of sophomores who shared a suite down the hall. One of the girls, Kathy, worked at a McDonald's up the road. On the nights when she covered the late shift and closed up shop, she and her coworkers were allowed to split any leftover burgers and fries, and take them home. My roommate and I would ask to be woken up when Kathy got home—usually between one and two in the morning—to get in on the booty. We'd stumble down to her suite and then sit bleary-eyed, shoving Big Macs or Filet-O-Fishes into our mouths. On nights when there wasn't enough for each of us to have our own, we'd pass the cold, rubbery excuses for food from person to person, taking a bite and handing it on, the way you'd pass a joint at a party. But it wasn't like a party at all. There was no music, no conversation. Only the sound of chewing, like a herd of cows grazing in a pasture.

We all laughed about those midnight munchies sessions, but they just added to the secret shame that continued to build as I piled on the pounds. I was ashamed of my thighs, my hips, my body. I was ashamed of my appetite, my driving need to stuff myself with anything and everything. But even more than that, I was ashamed of the powerlessness that kept me from saying "enough," that held me back from fully revealing the person I was inside and from reaching for the life I really wanted for myself. More than longing for the body of a super-model, I longed to live out loud—to feel free enough to liberate the woman hiding under all those layers of fleshy protective armor.

Yes, I know what it's like to feel trapped in your body and by your circumstances. To both love and hate the comfortable place you're in. I know how it is to be part of the scenery, to stand by, unseen, as all the things you want in life swirl around you, there for the taking, but you're too heavy to move. I know how it feels to want and hope, but be too afraid to act.

I know how it feels to be in the place you're in now. And I know the way out, too.

My Turning Point

After living the first twenty-five years or so of my life with the label Fat Girl, my weight peaked at around 185. I'm just under five feet four, so let's just say I didn't carry it well. It was back in the day when designer jeans had just come on the scene: Everybody, including me, wanted to get into some Calvins or Jordache or the cigarette-leg Guess jeans that were so impossibly tight they had zippers at the ankles so you could shimmy them over your feet. I was aching to trade in the double-pleated khakis that, rather than hiding my stomach and hips, made me look even more like one of Willy Wonka's Oompah Loompahs. I held on to that hope, only to find that even the largest size of Calvins (size 16) was too small for my ample butt.

By that time I had suffered so many defeats that I began to wonder why I dared to try anymore. Why take the jeans into the dressing room at all? I'd only end up back at the rack of "comfort-waist," "relaxed-fit" pants. Why pull out the dumbbell set collecting dust in the back of the closet? It would only remind me how physically and mentally weak I was as it sat there unused yet again. Why pass up my favorite bacon cheeseburger for a scantily dressed salad? The calories I'd save wouldn't make a dent in my weight. It was if I was trying to chip away at the U.S. deficit, one ten-cents-off coupon at a time.

I had so much to lose—and I'm not just talking about the weight. I stood to lose the life I knew, a life I wasn't happy in but one that was safe and comfortable. And yet I hated it. I hated always being the good girl, the giver, the one everyone could count on to pick up the slack, to get things done, but who was somehow always invisible. I hated how I constantly ignored my own needs and my own dreams, focusing instead on pleasing everyone around me, like a panting puppy just aching for a pat on the head. At the same time I was too afraid to let this life go. Deep down I knew that if I truly committed to changing, I wouldn't know what to do with myself. My legs were too heavy with fear to take the first step off that solid familiar platform onto the rickety makeshift bridge of "what if." I was afraid it would buckle under my weight, and I'd go crashing through to the hard ground beneath, unable to get back up again. But I was just as afraid I would manage to teeter and tiptoe to the other side—because I didn't know what awaited me there. For all my daydreaming, I simply couldn't imagine who I would be if I wasn't a Fat Girl anymore.

But one day something happened that made me want to find out.

The whole thing started with a half gallon of mint chocolate chip ice cream. I polished off the last third of the container, which I'd opened only the day before, straight from the carton.

As I shoveled the last of the ice cream into my mouth, though, my body decided it had had enough. A wave of nausea hit me, and I scrambled for the bathroom, barely making it to the toilet. At one point, mid-retch, I caught sight of myself in the mirror: bloated, pale, weak. Finally, I saw myself as I really was: powerless, full of shame, out of control, a victim of my appetite. And I vowed to do something about it.

I didn't quite believe that I could, but the reality of what I saw in the mirror that day gave me the strength to commit to trying. And that was the beginning of a journey that over the next three to five years revealed to me the body I was meant to have, and helped me discover the person I was meant to be.

Through lots of trial and lots of error, I finally managed to get my weight down to somewhere around 117, where I've kept it for the last twenty years or so. Along the way I reclaimed, recovered, and revealed the powerful, confident woman I am inside.

I was able to do what the so-called experts say is nearly impossible—what you no doubt think is impossible. I've been there. I know how it is to hear those success stories and think, "Good for you, girl. But I'm different. Just because *you* did it doesn't mean *I* can."

That's the way I used to think—that I was destined to be a

Fat Girl, that I was "big boned." I thought the girls I saw in the "before" and "after" shots were either fakes or had some kind of special willpower gene I wasn't born with.

But I'm no fake, no genetic mutant, and I'm not all that special, either. I just happened to stumble upon the solutions I needed as someone whose very identity was wrapped up in being a Fat Girl—someone whose specific needs weren't being addressed by the big-shot best seller diet gurus out there. While they were yammering about the details, such as how many carbs are too many carbs, whether dairy puts pounds on or takes them off, or which is better, low fat or low cal, they were completely ignoring the real issue. The real issue was not "How do I lose weight?" It was "How do I begin to think about myself as someone who *can* lose weight?"

Through my experience I'm convinced that being a Former Fat Girl is more about changing how you think about yourself and how you carry yourself in the world than what diet plan you're on or whose workout you follow. And that has implications far beyond the size of jeans you wear. It means that you are building the confidence that will allow you to be a success story in every aspect of your life, not just on the scale.

The measure of a Former Fat Girl isn't how many pounds you've lost, it's how you go for what you want in your life— how you take risks, speak up, and don't let fear or doubt rule you. It's how you walk through life with your chin up; how you look people in the eye when you speak.

The shift from wannabe Former Fat Girl to actual Former Fat Girl is about changing your life from the inside out, about going from seeing yourself as a victim of schoolyard nicknames and plus-size labels to a confident, secure, self-celebrating— and, yes, self-accepting—woman. It is about coming out of hiding and shedding the layers, both literally and figuratively, that prevent you from getting what you want out of life. Most of all, it is about identifying the obstacles in your way and finally having the support and resources to make the transition once and for all.

Your Starting Point

With my secrets and with my guidance you can make that transition. You can become a Former Fat Girl. You can harness the appetite that seems to control you. You can say no to unhealthy foods and unhealthy habits and mean it. You can break free of the fear and insecurity that hold you back from getting what you want in your life.

Even more than that, you can shed the image you carry around of yourself and start to see yourself in a new way. There is a place where you no longer have to hide all the things that make you special and unique, where you can let your personality shine and actually *flirt* if you so choose. As a Former Fat Girl, no longer will you have to bypass the cool clothes on your way to the "big girl" section of the department store. No longer will you be too ashamed to order crème brûlée, for fear that everyone in the restaurant will pity the poor Fat Girl who just can't deny her sweet tooth. No longer will you seek the comfort of the back row; you'll be the one on stage. You'll be the one who says what no one else has the courage to say. You'll be the first girl on the dance floor—with or without a partner.

I know you can get there, and I'm going to show you how. In this book I'll share the seven secrets I discovered on my journey to becoming a Former Fat Girl, the secrets I know will work for you, too. Along the way I'll reveal my struggles with the same issues you're facing, the issues that hold you back from having the body and the life you really deserve, from being the person, inside and out, you really are.

You might hate me now because I've done it and you're just getting started. You've had your hopes dashed many times before. But believe me when I say that you can do it. I know you can. I'll be with you all the way. Because if I could leave the past behind—with its broken chairs and stolen cookies and midnight McDonald's—you can, too.

Secrets of a Former Fat Girl

Chapter One

Secret #1: Forget Dieting

I didn't start out thinking I was doing anything revolutionary. Like most serial dieters, I had begun every other weight loss quest with a list of "no" foods—chocolate (of course) and desserts of any kind, butter, sugar, bread—all the things that made eating my favorite pastime and, it seemed, made life worth living.

But one day, on the heels of my ice cream–induced aha! moment, my friend Tracey (some names have been changed to protect the privacy of those individuals) invited me to her Jazzercise class, and, on a whim, I said yes. You know how it is: As many times as you might have failed in the past, you continue to have those flashes of hope that maybe this time things will be different. Maybe exercise won't be such a struggle; maybe you'll actually like it, like the skinny girls who hang out at the health club as if that were the most natural thing in the world.

If I had known what I was getting into, though, I probably would have stayed home. (Lesson #1: Ignorance can be a good thing.) Jazzercise was one of the early forms of aerobics—you know, back when Jane Fonda was feeling the burn in her leg warmers and matching headband. The class was part dance, part drill team routine set to the music of the time. I still remember part of the sequence to "What a Feeling" from the iconic 80s film *Flashdance*. One of the moves was derivative of John Travolta's signature *Saturday Night Fever* pose. We threw our hips to one side, jabbed our fingers into the air, and then switched to the other side on the frenzied beat. Thank God we didn't have camera phones back then.

At the time, I was a beleaguered graduate student in Austin, Texas. I had decided to go for my master's degree instead of getting a real job after college and was regretting my decision. I was tired of being a student; I felt as if I was in some kind of purgatory, waiting not so patiently for real life to begin. My life had stalled like my dilapidated four-door Datsun, and I needed some kind of push to get it going again. Before that flash of clarity on the bathroom floor, I would have told you that feeling was all about wanting to get out of school and start my career. But, looking back, I think it also had something to do with being stuck in a five-foot-four body that I had allowed to balloon up to 185 pounds—the heaviest I'd ever been.

Maybe that was why I said yes when Tracey suggested the class. Like me, Tracey was always on a diet, getting ready to go on a diet, or cheating on a diet. It was as if she and I were members of a secret sorority of Fat Girls (Thi Omega Phat?). We understood each other. We could joke about things we were too ashamed admit to anyone else—like the habit of eating while standing over the sink or at the refrigerator door or wearing your "fat pants" for the third day (or month or year) in a row.

I figured if Tracey had the nerve to squeeze into a leotard and cavort around with a bunch of strangers, maybe I could, too. And even if I did trip all over myself trying to keep up, at least I wouldn't be the only Fat Girl in the room. (Don't tell me you've never taken comfort in *that!*)

One problem: what to wear. It wasn't like my closet was full of cute little leotard and tights ensembles and I simply couldn't decide which to put on. Not only did I not own anything of the sort, but I couldn't imagine shoving my body into one. Hell, I could barely fit into everyday street clothes without a struggle. And this was back in the day, before you could go online and order anything you wanted under the radar (XXX videos? XXXL baby tees?) without having to worry about what the lady at the register might be thinking.

No, I would have to do what every Fat Girl absolutely dreads: go shopping.

At least my mother wasn't there. Mom and I had battled over my wardrobe since I was in fifth grade. That was in the early seventies when hip-huggers were hot and I was desperate to have a pair. I was desperate to have a pair because I was desperate to get in good with Susie, the coolest girl in the class, the girl who had already advanced beyond training bras, who sneaked smokes behind school, and who *really* knew what nasty words like *masturbation* meant when the boys made jokes about them instead of just playing along, like I did.

Shopping was horrible enough; shopping with Mom was excruciating for both of us. As gently as she could, Mom tried to steer me away from the low-slung crushed velour bell bottoms she knew would make me look as wide as a linebacker. I grabbed a pair and took them into the dressing room anyway, determined to prove her wrong—but, of course, I couldn't even button them over the folds of my stomach. You know the particular familiar pain. It wasn't just that the pants didn't fit—*I* didn't fit. I was never going to be "in" with Susie. I was never going to be anything more than part of the scenery, a Fat Girl who didn't deserve a spot in the inner circle. I sat in the dressing room for a while, unable to face my mom—not that she was the "I told you so" type, but she didn't need to be. Instead of accepting her support, crying on her shoulder, sharing my shame with her, I held it all in. I felt even more embarrassed knowing that she *knew*. It was completely lost on me in that moment—and in the many dressing room moments we would share in the future—that Mom and I shared the same body type. I know now that she had some of the very same struggles with her weight as I did, particularly when she was young. I don't think, though, that she experienced all the Fat Girl feelings I held inside. If she did, she'd have known how infuriating it was to see that look of pity in her eyes—infuriating because there was so much truth in it, truth I didn't want to face.

Thankfully, I would be the only one privy to my humiliation as I tried to find a leotard I could work my butt into without busting the seams. I drove to the discount store one weeknight, arriving just a half hour before closing time. I figured the place would be practically deserted, and the fewer customers who might raise their eyebrows at the chunky girl in the "activewear" section, the better.

One quick shuffle through the leotards on the rack was all it took, though, for me to decide not to buy one. I just couldn't face the prospect of trying the things on. It would be too much like swimsuit shopping, and you know how much fun that is. I picked up a package of tights from the sale bin, figuring I could wear them under a raggedy pair of polyester gym shorts from college. An XL T-shirt on top would be just fine; the more coverage, the better. If I could have worn a pup tent, I would have.

As I dressed for that first Jazzercise class, I realized the blinding pink tights I had bought were a mistake. There's a reason why road crews wear neon—the color practically screamed, "Get a load of these thighs!"

My worst fear was that, at the very sight of me, the other girls would laugh me out of the room. But that didn't happen.

The class instructor, Gina, was a tiny girl with exotic Asian looks and straight onyx hair down to her perfect little butt. She was funny and not too perky (I hate perky), and didn't recoil in horror, drop to the floor laughing, or say, "Sorry. Overeaters Anonymous meets down the hall," when I walked into class. In fact, she didn't seem to look at me any differently than any of the other women in the room—who, by the way, weren't exactly anatomically perfect specimens, either. I secretly studied them all, Gina included, looking for any sign that they were judging me. If I had picked up on any "thinner than thou" vibes, I would never have gone back.

Class was at an Episcopal church near campus, in a linoleum-floored room probably used for coffee and doughnut socials after Sunday services. Wood paneling covered three of the walls; on the fourth, behind the small, carpeted podium where Gina perched, was a mirror the width of the room. Thank God there were still spots in the back row, or I'd have had a full frontal view of myself the entire class. It was bad enough that wherever I stood, I couldn't get away from my reflection. I kept trying to duck behind the skinny girl in front of me until she noticed and gave me a look.

But when Gina put the music on and began to move, I soon became so caught up in watching her that I didn't give my image more than a passing glance during the forty-minute class. It was really a matter of self-defense: If I didn't pay attention, I'd end up grapevining left when everyone else was going right and cause an ugly pileup. And while that didn't happen, I still screwed up, making a mess of the simple choreography to a Pointer Sisters tune. But I wasn't the only one. And something about the way Gina handled it—as if it were no big deal, as if the point of the whole thing was to keep moving and not worry about doing it perfectly—made screwing up less than mortifying. She did laugh, but the way she laughed made me laugh, too, and I wasn't the type to laugh at myself very easily.

Something else happened, something I didn't quite expect. As I started to focus on moving with her, I forgot for just a little while that I was a Fat Girl who had no business being there. In that forty-minute period, my self-consciousness took a backseat as I concentrated on what I was doing and not on how I looked while I was doing it. The flash of hope that got me to that Jazzercise class in the first place ignited something in me. The idea began to flicker in my mind that maybe I could do it. I could move. I could dance. I could sweat. I could *exercise*.

I didn't know it then, but this time *would* prove to be different.

I started going to Jazzercise regularly, chasing the "I can" feeling it gave me—a feeling I had never gotten during any of my many previous weight loss ventures. Mostly, I'd tried to manage my weight the "no" way—no dessert, no bread, no butter, no, no, no. Exercise had been an exercise in frustration. I had tried running in high school, sustaining a routine (if you could call it that) for a couple of weeks at a time. But I could never get my breathing right and never felt comfortable physically or emotionally. I concluded that I wasn't the athletic type. After all, how many Fat Girls do you see at the Olympics?

I brought my workout bag with me to campus every Monday, Wednesday, and Friday so I could go straight from my part-time job. It wasn't something I looked forward to exactly; it was something I just *did*, like some women meet girlfriends for lunch or drinks. In that way, Jazzercise became my social life. I didn't gab much with the other women in the class or anything, but I did feel some kind of connection with them. And, of course, it was a place to meet up with Tracey.

I know that part of the reason I became such a faithful Jazzercizer was out of shame. The last thing I wanted to do was skip class and have people think I wimped out, that I was slacking. For once my Fat Girl programming was working for me. It was the people-pleasing perfectionist inside of me that wouldn't let me quit. But when I couldn't make it for a legitimate reason— a trip to visit my family in Houston, for instance—I found that I actually missed it. Amazing. Who would have thought that I'd ever be hooked on anything more strenuous than wrestling the lid off a half gallon of mint chocolate chip?

Jazzercise proved to be my gateway drug. It led the way to stiffer stuff—specifically, to running. The minor flirtation I had with running in high school came at a time when I was particularly determined to do something about my weight. But like previous forays into fitness, that one lasted about as long as a bag of M&Ms in my kitchen cabinet.

Five Former Fat Girl Wardrobe Basics to Get You Started

Isn't it ironic that we have to wear revealing clothing in order to get in shape so we feel confident in revealing clothing? A conundrum for wannabe Former Fat Girls for sure. Here are five easy solutions that will minimize the embarrassment and make you more comfortable and confident:

1. **Basic black pants.** Always slimming, always easy. Slightly thicker, moisture-wicking fabric will help smooth you out a bit. A lower rise (just under your navel) and a boot-cut silhouette will be flattering and allow you to move with ease. Use these as your staples. I suggest getting at least two pairs, maybe more depending on how often you do laundry.

2. **Technical tees.** Tops made of so-called technical fabrics— synthetic blends such as Coolmax—really do help keep you cooler and more comfortable during a workout. They are designed to move the sweat away from the skin to the surface of the fabric where it will evaporate. They are available from most makers (try activa.com and titlenine.com) in both loose and fitted styles.

3. **A light jacket.** Something to throw on when you're going to and from the gym or to keep you warm on an early-morning

walk. Again, choose a technical fabric to help disperse and evaporate moisture. A style that hits just below your bottom and cinches a bit at the waist will not only be more flattering than a shorter style but also will help keep your butt covered in cool weather.

4. **Socks.** Cotton socks are a big no-no. They trap moisture, leading to blisters and ugly athlete's foot. It's better to invest in pairs made of synthetic moisture-wicking blends. Look for styles made for your particular activity, because the construction and padding will be different for a walker, for instance, than it would be for a cyclist. Also, be sure to bring your socks when you're trying on a pair of shoes; you want to be sure the two feel right together.

5. **Underwear.** It's no use investing in pants made of technical fabrics if you're wearing cotton or nylon underneath. Panties that do just as good a job of wicking sweat are widely available from brands like Champion and from activa.com and titlenine.com. Not only is that a comfort issue, but it could be a health issue as well: Yeast infections thrive in warm, sweaty environments. Plus, these fabrics have a lot of give, so you'll be able to move through your workout with ease.

What would become my last best attempt to be a runner, the one that stuck, began on an almost abandoned quarter-mile dirt track. I drove there one evening at dusk in the same tights-with-gym-shorts getup I had squeezed myself into for Jazzercise. What made me do it that night, I don't really know. Maybe I wasn't getting the same feeling out of "What a Feeling" as I had those first several months of class. I do know that without the strength (mental, not so much physical) I had built in Jazzercise, I would never have taken that first step. Jazzercise had helped me open my mind just a little bit to the idea that maybe I could change, maybe I didn't have to be stuck, maybe I could shed the Fat Girl image that had defined me for so long.

I set out to run just one lap. I pounded through it, surging and then flagging without much rhythm. It felt odd, hard, but not odd enough or hard enough for me to give up. I tried another. I did a quick body check: Nothing was broken. I hadn't had a coronary; my lungs hadn't exploded. I glanced around: There were no horrified onlookers. So—what the hell—I ran a third. I made it through four laps that night. That's a mile, mind you. A *mile*. On a *track*. Where *runners* belong—not people like me.

Strange, though. Rather than feeling like a trespasser, I was a little thrilled. I did it. I, the Fat Girl, ran a mile! I was flushed with not just exertion but with the kind of sensation you get after you do something out of character and risky, like blurting out how you really feel about a crush and not caring at that moment whether he feels the same way.

The rush faded, though, overpowered by the loud complaining from my body over what I had just put it through. My feet hurt, my legs tingled. This was nothing like Jazzercise.

But still I wanted more. If Jazzercise had given me that "I can" feeling, running did even more. After all, it was more *athletic*, something only strong, slim girls did. I went back to the track two nights later and two nights after that to run in the cool cover of dark.

Don't get me wrong. It was hard. It was hard every night, physically—the pounding on my poor hips, knees, and feet (in particular the bunions I had inherited from Grandmom). It was especially hard to find the energy to do anything more than make it up the three flights to my apartment.

It was even harder mentally to get myself into my running clothes and to that track, and then to slog through lap after lap after lap. Despite the rush that running gave me, I had years of Fat Girl programming to fight against: all those feelings that told me I didn't belong, that I couldn't do it—the powerlessness, the temptation to stay in that comfortable, miserable place I had known for so long. As much as I wanted to break out and let the woman inside shine, I was afraid.

That fear bubbled up in different ways all through the day, mostly in the form of something I call my "inner whiner." That's the little voice you have in your head that brings up every possible excuse for not exercising. "It's too hard." "It's *sooooo* hot outside!" "You'll mess up your hair."

I came up with all kinds of tricks to help combat that fear. For instance, I found that it was especially difficult to get my butt to the track if I went home to change first. When I did, I had to fight off the urge to curl up on the couch and watch TV instead. Why waste the energy? I needed every bit to get me through the run itself. So I started carrying my workout bag with me, going straight to the track and changing in a restroom there.

I also devised some mind games to make running more tolerable. I had this particular way of counting laps. If I was trying to run six laps total, I'd divide the number in half—

three, in this case. When I finished the first lap, I'd say (in my head; I'm not that weird), "Two more to halfway." After the next lap it was "One more to halfway." After lap three I'd say, "Three more to the finish." I'd repeat those phrases over and over as I ran, trying to drown out the voice of that inner whiner who was always asking, "Can we stop now, *pleeeeeeze?*"

Until then my imagination was the only thing about me that you could call active. Now I put to use the skills I honed creating elaborate daydreams about marrying the latest teen idol (Davy Jones of the Monkees was an early favorite). Some nights at the track I'd visualize myself running before a roaring crowd, slogging toward the finish line. I'd break the imaginary tape, and after looking around to make sure I wasn't being watched, I'd raise both hands in victory. Yeah, I can't believe I did something so corny, either. But it had become a matter of survival. I was ready to do whatever it took to get to the end of that run, to win.

That's how I felt after every track session: a little more like a winner. Running did something for me that Jazzercise didn't. Each lap I completed was an instant success, a task I'd checked off my to-do list. For the overachiever in me, it was like a drug. I needed more. Each lap was a goal I could tick off before moving on to the next. I worked my way up to running a mile and a half, then two, then three. The way I felt after a run—not physically but emotionally—dulled the soreness in my muscles, the aches in my bunions. Every time I inched a bit farther than before, I felt like an explorer breaking new ground. What I was doing was as impossible to me as it was for Neil Armstrong to walk on the moon or Keanu Reeves to do Shakespeare. I ran on that track exclusively for at least a year, spurred on by the strokes I got from finishing lap after lap.

* * *

In the meantime, I was still up to my old dietary indiscretions, the ones that compelled me to polish off a supersize order of fries or an entire sleeve of Girl Scout cookies even though I knew I'd be doubled over in pain afterward. My favorite dinner at the time—my post-run reward—was a homemade ground beef soft taco piled with cheese, guacamole, and sour cream. Not exactly what you'd call light. Dessert was a pint of cookies and cream ice cream. (Okay, so I had downsized a bit from my usual half gallon.)

Unbelievably, despite my food free-for-alls, I started losing weight. My waistbands started feeling looser, my thighs not as loose. After several months I was out of my fattest-of-fat pants and into my somewhat-less-fat pants. I went down a couple of sizes, from a 16 or so to a 12, *without changing the way I was eating at all.*

I was no dummy. I knew exercise could burn off some of the junk a person eats. But I had never experienced it myself. I mean, I was eating ice cream by the pint several days a week, and *still* my body was changing. Amazing!

The more weight I lost, the easier running became and the more I wanted to do it. I could see and feel the difference physically. The three flights up to my apartment didn't leave me puffing like an old-lady smoker. Even shopping for clothes began to be less painful. I could actually find pieces that fit, though I stayed far away from leotards, swimsuits, and, of course, jeans.

I loved what running was doing to my body, but at first I took the weight loss in stride. After all, I had been there before. I had lost my share of pounds at other times in my life, only to gain them back. I didn't quite trust it. Not yet.

The small flicker of hope that got me to Jazzercise in the first place continued to burn, and burn brighter, but it wasn't

Club Dread: The Former Fat Girl's Cure

Back in my old pre-Jazzercise days, the thought of stepping into a health club made me want to reach for the Tums. But there are places where buns of steel and showgirl cleavage aren't part of the membership requirements. Take a tour, try a class, and see for yourself at these health clubs:

- **The YMCA.** At my Y, where I have been a member for more than ten years, I see ex-college football players working out alongside ninety-one-year-old great-grandmas. There is always an amazing slice of life no matter what Y you visit.

- **Community fitness centers.** These are very family oriented and less likely to be on the singles pick-up circuit.

- **Churches.** How intimidating can the coffee and doughnuts room at the Episcopal church be? (I had been there many times for the doughnuts before I discovered Jazzercise.) More and more churches are including yoga and other fitness classes in their schedules. And who knows, you might get some points in the spiritual department, too.

- **Women-only gyms.** We know that girls can be just as brutal as men (if not more), but women-only health clubs often attract women who aren't there to attract men. I don't know about you, but I have a hard time feeling good about myself in my husband's old running shorts when I'm surrounded by women who look like they should be bar-hopping on a Saturday night. Some women-only clubs, like the Curves chain, specifically focus on minimizing the intimidation factor for their members.

- **Private training.** Depending on your personality and budget, working out with a trainer in a private studio—where it's just you and her (and I would go with a *her*)—might be the way to go. Of course, that's the priciest option here, but the size of the check you write can be a powerful motivator. (They cash the check whether you show up or not, so you'd better go to make it worthwhile.)

connected as much to the weight I was dropping. In fact, I wasn't really focused on the pounds I was losing at all. I didn't even weigh myself. All I thought about was running, how to get through the eight or ten laps I had to do that day and how many I might be able to run tomorrow. I was chasing that "I can" feeling I first got from Jazzercise and felt even stronger from running. I was exercising for the positive things it was doing for my mind and my body, not to work off the bag of chips I had at lunch.

And that, I know now, is what really made the difference this time: my single-minded focus on exercise. Exercise did two things for me: It helped me begin to break through the image I had of myself as a Fat Girl, and it fed me the encouraging, motivating, "I can" messages I needed at the beginning of this process.

I realized that because most diets emphasize what you're eating—or, more specifically, what you shouldn't be eating—they are doomed to fail. They are all about "You can't" and "You shouldn't."

Oh, sure, I lost at least a few pounds every time I tried a new program, but the problem was that I loved food. I didn't just love to eat it. I loved everything about it—making it, shopping for it, reading about it. Telling me I couldn't eat the stuff I loved was like trying to keep a teenage girl away from her bad-apple boyfriend—down to the deception she would use to hook up with him anyway. I was trying to deny myself one of the things I enjoyed most, and it just plain didn't feel good. I was a failure because I couldn't control my appetite. I couldn't live without chocolate or pasta or burgers and fries, at least not for more than a couple of weeks. I was so frustrated by all my attempts at dieting that I really didn't believe I could ever succeed. I felt weak. I wanted to hide. I didn't know if I had the will to even try again.

What I needed, I know now, was an infusion of power, and I got it when I started exercising. Instead of saying no, no, no to my appetite, exercise was all about saying yes, saying I can, feeling the power of pushing myself further than I ever had—even if it was to the music of *Flashdance* while wearing a lumpy leotard. It fed my ego, the only part of me (except maybe my cup size) that needed any kind of enhancement. I began to crave that feeling of personal power almost as much as a Hershey's bar. Almost.

And that, dear future Former Fat Girls, is why I've made Forget Dieting secret number one. The subtext could be Start Moving because to begin your transformation you need to start feeling like a winner. You need to start chipping away at the idea that you are powerless, weak, stuck. Exercise can be the answer if you do it like a Former Fat Girl. Read on to find out how.

Move Like a Former Fat Girl

Okay, so you're starting to get it: This isn't some garden-variety diet. For one thing, how many weight loss plans start by giving you permission to forget about what you're eating (or trying not to eat)? You're probably used to those diets that from the very start expect you to cut back drastically on the foods you love and crave. I know how hard that is and how bad it feels to constantly tell yourself no, I can't, I shouldn't.

Cleaning out the vending machine every afternoon is not okay just because you walk on the treadmill every morning. But to begin to see yourself as a Former Fat Girl, you have to work on making exercise as much of a habit as your 3:00 P.M.

snack attack. Conquering the treadmill, the track, the pool, whatever, is going to help you reimagine yourself more than any old diet would, and that's the real work that has to happen if you are to become a Former Fat Girl.

Nor is this the same old advice about how to start an exercise program. What's different about my approach is that it focuses on exercise as the starting point in your quest for Former Fat Girldom because of what it does for your *mind*. It sets you up for life-changing success by helping you flip that switch in your head to the "I can" position. As you make exercise a regular habit, as much a part of your life as brushing and flossing (okay, so maybe more regular than flossing), you begin to feed your self-confidence bit by bit. You start peeling away that Fat Girl label you've lived with and start allowing that vibrant, worthy Former Fat Girl to emerge.

I know that for you exercise isn't just a matter of slipping on your sneakers and going to the gym. Just finding workout clothes and shoes that fit your body and your needs, for instance, is a challenge—not to mention all the emotional issues that bubble up. There's the pounding, the bouncing, the soreness, the equipment you don't know how to use. I know what it's like to walk into a fitness class or step onto a running track and feel like an outsider, like some geeky kid crashing the cool crowd's party.

Compared to that, dieting might seem easy, as simple as scratching out things on your grocery list and replacing them with stuff that doesn't have high-fructose corn syrup, partially hydrogenated oils, and rendered animal fat at the top of their ingredients lists. But it is such a negative, spirit-sucking way to live. You, future Former Fat Girl, need all the strokes you can get, especially at the beginning. Think of exercise as the first chapter of your success story, because it will help you build a stockpile of personal power and steel you for the rest of the journey ahead. The making-better-food-choices bit will come later.

Here are my secrets for getting over, around, and through those obstacles and moving toward life as a Former Fat Girl.

The Obstacle: The Whiner in Your Head

My whiner, whom you've already met, would pipe up whenever she had the opportunity: "Do we *really* have to run today?" Or "My toe is hurting. Can't we stop now?" Sometimes, desperate to get my attention, she turned just plain nasty: "Who are *you* to think you can be a runner, fatty?" I tried to figure out when I heard her most clearly and then devised clever little tactics to shut her up. Here's what helped me.

Former Fat Girl Fixes

Don't exercise at home.

Show me a person who actually uses the treadmill in her bedroom, and I'll show you ten who walk over it, around it, or anywhere but *on* it. Why? Because they give in to the whiner who astutely points out all the other things you could (that is, *should*) be doing instead of logging those miles, doing those crunches, or folding yourself into that downward dog. Like cleaning out your cosmetics case, dusting the ceiling fan, or writing a note to that woman—what was her name? The one you worked with three career moves ago. She was great, wasn't she? All those good times you had . . .

See how the whiner distracts! Wily little thing. If you were at a gym or the Y or the community pool or track, you'd be among other people avoiding their own whiners and not surrounded by your clutter, your couch, your computer, or in close proximity to your pantry. Oh, the whiner would still be there, and she could still talk you into cutting your workout short. It may be pride or ego, but I find it hard to walk out of the weight room or the kickboxing class after only ten minutes or so. It just doesn't seem worth the trouble.

You may feel as welcome at a health club as you would in a men's restroom, so working out at home to a video or on a treadmill might seem like a good way to avoid the whole scene. But at home it's too easy to give into your inner whiner and end up on the couch watching *Wheel of Fortune* and struggling to ignore the bag of Doritos calling you from the pantry. And even if you do prefer to exercise outside, you definitely need an indoor option. One of the whiner's favorite things to bellyache about is the weather. "You want to go out in *this*? It's too ccccccold." Or "You won't be satisfied until I die of heat stroke."

Where, then, can you go to sweat without feeling like an alien? A good place to start are walking trails and high school or college tracks (after practice, of course; the last thing you want to do is get run over by a bunch of long-legged coeds with zero body fat). If you are shopping for a club, check out the YMCA. The best Ys offer cutting-edge fitness programs and equipment, a family-friendly vibe, and very few Lycra thongs. You are more likely to see girls (and guys) of all shapes, sizes, and ages there than you would at the "hot" clubs in town. Finally, a growing recognition among the health club industry of the fear factor among beginners and women in particular has spawned the growth of women's-only fitness chains. These clubs, such as Curves, use small classes and personalized attention to help you overcome your intimidation. (For more on getting past your "club dread," see the sidebar on page 14.)

Make it as convenient as possible.

You want to do all you can to get rid of any excuses that might set off the whiner in your head, so when you're considering where you want to work out, factor in location. I suggest finding a place that's on your way to or from somewhere you go several times a week—like work, or your kids' school. The more convenient it is for you, the better. It gives the whiner less ammunition (no "But it's so far a*waaaaaaaay*").

It's better for the gym or Y or whatever you choose to be closer to your destination than to your house, or you might be tempted to stop off and change before your workouts. That's just another opportunity for your whiner to remind you how nice it would be to settle down and unwind for "just a minute" on that soft, pillowy couch before going to that "horrible, nasty" place to sweat.

This means, of course, that you have to have somewhere to get dressed, most probably a locker room among lots of sweaty or soon-to-be sweaty women in various stages of undress. You might have no problem with this, but back in my fat days, I was terrified at the very idea of getting naked with a bunch of strangers. I could barely stand to get naked with myself. I came up with an admittedly imperfect solution—imperfect because not only would it offend Ms. Manners's sensibilities but because it might also be actionable in some states. In direct violation of the rules of gym etiquette, I'd sneak my stuff into a bathroom stall and change there—sometimes, I admit, in the one reserved for disabled women. I was always very quick and never came out to find a line of women in wheelchairs glaring at me.

I've also seen fully dressed women lug their workout bags right into a curtained shower stall to change, which is also probably frowned upon. But you gotta do what you gotta do.

After a while you'll begin to get over yourself. I've become so uninhibited that I'm afraid someday I'll forget and walk out topless into a common area for an extra towel. Part of the reason, of course, is that I'm not carrying around an extra seventy pounds of flab anymore. But what really helped cure my locker room phobia was the sight of other women who seemed not to mind that their bodies were less than perfect. One scene still runs through my head: In the locker room at the Y in Chapel Hill, North Carolina, where I lived for a brief time several years ago, there was a fifty-something woman bearing the scars of a double mastectomy; another the age of my mom, all folds of crepelike skin, coming in from her swim; another a UNC student who looked to be battling the "freshman fifteen"; and me. All different bodies, all imperfect, all naked, all getting stronger, feeling more powerful, and doing right by themselves. It was just another day in the locker room, but for me there was a feeling that we were all in this together. There was no self-consciousness, no scrutiny, no judgments, only acceptance.

Until it is no big deal to you, do what you have to do to make yourself comfortable. The women around you know what you're going through, believe me. And if they don't, well, you can probably imagine what I'd tell them (or at least think to myself).

Drown her out.

Remember the Rain Man–like way I used to count laps ("two more to halfway," "one more to halfway")? Not only did that help keep me from cheating myself out of a lap or two, which I was always tempted to do at first, but it gave me something to think about, something other than the voice in my head kvetching about my aching knees and cramping muscles. An easier way to drown out the whiner, though, is with music. Once I graduated from the track to a trail—one long, continuous loop where counting just didn't make sense—I couldn't live without my Walkman. (Remember them? They were the iPods of the 80s and 90s.) If you're one of the three people in the world who doesn't have an MP3 player, get one. They're cheap—under $100—and even a computerphobe like me can program one. (Or, for a little fun, you can hand yours over to your husband, a friend, or even a teenager if you're daring, to download away.) A little music will make your workout more tolerable. There are safety issues if you exercise outdoors with headphones on: When you're bopping along to the booming bass of Usher, you might not hear an approaching car or footsteps behind you. Not to be paranoid or anything, but I have a good tip from running coach Jenny Hadfield (who holds beginner running clinics for women called Run Like a Girl). She suggests using only one earpiece, leaving the other ear on alert.

If you're into the treadmill, stationary bike, or elliptical trainer, try watching TV, but make sure what you're watching is something you really want to watch and not just whatever junk happens to be on at the time. For instance, tape or TiVo a favorite show you never get to see (I find the *E! True Hollywood Stories* are fabulous for this) and allow yourself to watch it only while you're working out. That'll give you something to look forward to and something more likely to divert your attention from the whiner.

Delegate the details.

Hmmm. Should I exercise Monday, Wednesday, and Friday? Or Tuesday and Thursday? Early morning, mid-morning, after work? These details may seem insignificant, but they're perfect opportunities for the whiner to step in and say, "Exercise is too much trouble. Too many decisions. Let's just forget it."

There are a couple of ways to dispense with such details. One is to find a class, as I did with Jazzercise. It wasn't up to me to decide what time to exercise or how often; there was a set schedule to follow. I didn't have to entertain myself during class; I could leave that to the teacher, my classmates, and (obscure disco reference alert) Gloria Gaynor.

Another is to find a walking or running group. That may not be as hard as you think: YMCAs, neighborhood centers, and even fitness footwear stores and employers often have groups that tend to be pretty low-commitment. All you do is show up at the appointed time and place, and you're in.

The problem with both of these approaches, of course, is that you have to be somewhat of a joiner to take the first step. But remember: I wasn't exactly what you'd call the social type. If you're a loner, as I was, or you just don't feel good enough about yourself to be all chatty with a group of strangers, a class might be better for you. After all, you can't exactly be expected to share the details of your life over the thumping from the sound system. And everyone is usually focusing on trying to get the movements down, so there's really not much opportunity to share recipes or anything.

The walking and running group types, on the other hand, tend to gab to help pass the time while they lope along. (Some people do have the lung capacity to talk and run simultaneously!) If you go that route and want to keep to yourself, here's my advice: Exchange a few pleasantries during warm-up stretches so that people know you're not a total jerk, then strap on your MP3 player and go. I doubt you'll offend anyone.

Stay workout ready.

One of those details you can't delegate but that will give your whiner one less thing to gripe about is keeping your workout clothes clean and your bag packed and ready to go. First things first: Make sure you have enough sets of fitness clothes to get you from wash day to wash day. That way you'll never get caught without a clean pair of shorts or bra the morning of a workout. (No excuses!)

Second, the workout bag. If you're following this Former Fat Girl's advice, you'll be changing somewhere besides your own home, so you'll need to carry your clothes with you. To save you from packing and repacking completely the night before or the morning of every workout, keep whatever you can in your bag at all times—your shoes, for one, and any toiletries you might need to freshen up afterward. The minute you get home from one workout, swap out your dirty duds with a complete set of clean ones; then you won't have to rummage around for a runaway sock or a decent T-shirt when you're in a hurry.

The Obstacle: Exercise Just Plain Hurts

Have I mentioned my bunions? If you're lucky enough not to have them or even know what they are, let me explain. Bunions are bony knobs located on the side of your foot, at the base of your big toe. Not only are they particularly unattractive (I've said in the past that I'd rather show my bare ass than my bare feet), but they tend to throb after long periods of standing. Repeated jumping or pounding? I've been known to snack on Advil like it was popcorn to get a little post-workout relief. I know pain, and I've figured out several ways of keeping it to a minimum.

Former Fat Girl Fixes

Forget "no pain, no gain."

It's tempting to throw yourself into the type of workout that's going to give you the maximum calorie burn in the minimum amount of time. You have so much too lose, you think, and you want to lose it as fast as you can. Remember, though, that this is all about building an exercise habit you can live with. It's about changing your life for good, not just getting to some number on the scale. You are in this to become the kind of person for whom exercise is second nature. You're not going to do it for three months, six months, a year, and then give it up.

Even if you have dipped into more strenuous forms of exercise in the past, like I did before latching onto the gentler Jazzercise, it's better to start with something that's easy on your body, something you will more likely stay with and succeed at. Starting soft and slow will help you build that fitness habit every Former Fat Girl must have. And it will lay the physical groundwork for the more intense forms of fitness you may want to get into later. Activities such as yoga, Pilates, water aerobics, swimming, and stationary cycling are all low-impact exercises that give you a great workout but are easier on your body. You'll still be burning calories and getting stronger, but you're less likely to struggle or to overdo it and end up with an injury. I can tell you from personal experience how devastating it is to get all juiced up about an exercise program and then get smacked down by a sprained ankle, sore knee, or aching back. So-called overuse injuries—aches and pains from overdoing it—are some of the main reasons that women (and men) give up exercise altogether. All the more reason to take time to build up your strength and stamina.

Dress for success.

If you're into it, go ahead and spring for a complete color-coordinated workout wardrobe. But if you're like I was, the last thing you want to do is shop. Whatever you end up doing, though, make sure you invest some time and money in two key accessories: shoes and bras.

Shoes were big for me, bunions and all, but a good pair of fitness shoes is essential even for women with sleek, perfect feet. Unless you're involved in a zero-impact exercise, like swimming or yoga (which you do barefoot), the right shoes can make your entire workout easier on your body. Take the knees, for example. Achy knees are one of the plagues of beginning runners and walkers—especially women who take up the sport to try to lose weight. A good cushy-yet-supportive pair can help insulate your knees from some of the pounding. Many of the major shoe companies—New Balance, Saucony, Asics, and Rykä (which makes only women's fitness shoes)—even offer walking and running models for "heavy" runners. You might want to start there if your sneakers tend to break down quickly. (Trust me, you'll need them only in the beginning.)

As for the bra issue, I recently read that the average cup size of the American woman is a D. Just another thing I'm way below average on: If they made a negative A, that would be me. But back in my bigger days, I had my share of breast tissue, so I can relate. Plus, I've talked with many women about the pain they feel in their chests, backs, and shoulders when they attempt even low-impact exercise like walking, and the frustration of finding a bra that will keep "the girls" tethered without feeling as if they're in a straitjacket.

The bouncing boob issue is another reason to start with a gentle, low-jiggle form of exercise. Even so, you'll still need

Bra Basics: Keeping the Girls Comfy

I am so flat that I could probably do all my bra shopping in the preteen department. Comfort and support are still important for women like me, but for those who are more on the average and above-average side (cupwise, I mean), they are crucial. Here's the Former Fat Girl's guide to finding a fitness bra that will give you both.

- **Allow for the impact factor.** Possibly the most important thing to consider is where your typical type of workout falls on the impact scale. Is it high, low, or somewhere in between? Most manufacturers and many catalogs and Web sites rate their bras by the level of impact they can withstand. Activa (www.activasports.com) and Title Nine (www.titlenine.com) are two of the best.

- **Pick a sweat-wicking fabric.** Fabrics such as Coolmax, Nike's Dry-FIT, and Champion's DoubleDry work to move moisture away from your body so your skin stays drier. Your bra will be less likely to rub you the wrong way if your skin is dry.

- **Go seamless.** No seams mean less chafing: Brands such as Champion and Nike offer a variety of seamless models, some of them with underwire construction.

- **Look for wider, padded straps.** Wider straps help distribute the load (sorry!) more evenly to ease the strain on your shoulders. Some bras use gel in the straps for an even comfier ride.

- **Choose a model with molded cups.** This kind of bra lifts and supports while maintaining your girlish shape. Virtually shapeless "compression" bras, on the other hand, use sheer force. You might as well duct tape them down.

- **Get some advice.** You'd be amazed at how detailed some of the apparel Web sites are; for instance, Activa gives recommendations for specific bras that address particular problems and walks you step by step through the process of taking your measurements. The site also offers a toll-free number in case you can't find the info you need or just want to chat. The women at Title Nine have a sense of humor about what they do, and it shows. They call their bras things like the Wired and Ready for Action Bra and (my favorite) The Last Resort Bra, their recommendation for the big, bouncy girl who has tried every other bra out there.

something to wear up top. The good news is that the fitness apparel industry is no longer ignoring women whose breasts are bigger than an eleven-year-old's. You'll get the best selection online (see the sidebar on page 28 for details), but you're better off trying on a few different styles to get a feel for what you like. Some major brands (such as Champion) offer sizes up to DD and are carried in major department stores like Macy's and Nordstrom. Innovations such as gel straps, contoured cups, and front closures can help you get a comfortable fit even for high-impact activities like running.

Follow the 10 percent rule.

For anyone who exercises—from the elite athlete to the wannabe Former Fat Girl—any workout will get easier after about six weeks of doing it regularly. That means two things: To keep getting stronger, burn more calories, and lose more weight, you have to push yourself even harder, but in your excitement at your progress or your anxiousness to keep the results coming, you may push so hard that you hurt yourself. The last thing you want to do is get on a roll, and—bam!—end up nursing a sore knee, an achy ankle, or worse.

That's where the 10 percent rule comes in. It's used by trainers and other experts to help you figure out how to keep pushing yourself without going too far. It goes like this: Each week you are allowed to increase the intensity, distance, or difficulty level of your workout by a maximum of 10 percent. That means if you're walking two miles this week and feel up to it, you can add .8 of a lap next week. Round it up to make it easier to keep track of. Or if you're walking your two miles in, say, thirty minutes, try to pick up your pace to shave off three minutes. That doesn't seem like much, I know, but it will when you try to do it.

Step away from the mirror.

The reason for the wall-to-wall mirrors in most workout rooms isn't to fuel the vanity of girls in outfits who look as if they came straight from their waitressing jobs at Hooters. Nor are they meant to torture everyone else with the sight of their soft middles and muscles. The real reason for them is to allow people who know what they're looking for to monitor their form and to give you a 360-degree view of the instructor during class.

But there is a downside to staring at yourself in the mirror if you're new to the whole workout scene. An interesting study suggests that watching yourself move your body in unfamiliar ways might actually make you feel as if you're working harder than you actually are. This is not a good thing when you're on a quest for Former Fat Girlhood and trying to get into (or get back into) the habit of exercising. It is better to claim a spot a couple of rows back in your fitness class. (Most probably the class veterans and guys lusting after the teacher will nab the first rows anyway.) As for the cardio and weight rooms, if you can't find a mirrorless spot, try looking at the TV or focusing on the floor or ceiling. If you're doing a weight move or riding a stationary bike, close your eyes.

The Obstacle: You Don't Like Exercise

I know what you mean. For a long time I thought there must be an "I love exercise" gene that I don't have. And maybe there is—right next to the "never a bad hair day" gene or the "eat chocolate, lose weight" gene. Until modern science discovers them and figures out how to put their powers in a pill, we all have to deal. Here are my tactics.

Shoes Rule: How to Find the Right Fit

Every so often some group of podiatrists releases a survey showing that some amazing percentage of women are walking around at any given moment in shoes that don't fit. I'm not going to go into the reasons that that's true; let's just say we women are notorious for having trouble sizing things up.

This isn't a mere comfort issue for women on the heavy side who are just starting to get active. The wrong pair of fitness shoes can sidetrack you on your way to becoming a Former Fat Girl. Here is how not to let that happen.

- Match the shoe to the activity you do regularly. If you're a runner, you should buy a pair of running shoes; if you're a walker, walking shoes. It's really not some evil marketing ploy to get you to spend money on a closet full of fitness shoes. Shoes for different activities feature different technologies; for instance, walking shoes are more flexible under the ball of your foot than running shoes to accommodate the rolling and pushing off you do.

- Think about your feet. Are they wide like mine, and do you have high arches or narrow heels? Certain manufacturers and Web sites can help you match styles to the shape of your foot. Brands that are particularly good for women include New Balance and Asics, both of which come in different widths, and Rykä, which makes only women's shoes and is particularly good for walking, cross training, or studio shoes.

- Try a style built for "heavy runners" if running is your activity of choice. Okay, so the hope is that you won't need this particular piece of advice for long. But shoe companies—from Avia to Asics to Rykä as well as New Balance and Saucony—in the last couple of years have introduced models specifically for women who are hard on their shoes. They typically have more support and are less flexible, and therefore stand up better to the pounding paces you put them through.

- Know how you move. Certain shoes are constructed to compensate for issues you might have with your stride. The most common is the tendency to roll inward (called pronation). The easiest way to figure out if that is an issue for you is to look at a pair of athletic shoes or flats in your closet. Look at the soles for any signs of wear. If the cushioning is broken down or the tread is worn away along the inner edges of the balls of your feet, you're probably a pronator. Shoes with what is called "motion control" can help correct that problem and make your activity more comfortable.

- Specialty shop. Why shop in person when you can get anything you want on the Internet (without the humiliation of being waited on by skinnier-than-thou salespeople)? Because as well as you know shoes and as hard as you try to match your foot to them, you really have to try them on before you buy. If they don't feel good the minute you put them on your feet, they're not going to after standing up and walking around. Forget the whole "breaking in" bit.

Don't expect to love it.

Here's a little secret: I don't particularly like to exercise—especially running, and I've put in a lot of miles over the last twenty years. I meet people all the time who tell me they've just started running and are working at it, but they just can't wait to experience the "runner's high" they've heard so much about. Well, I've run ten marathons, and I think I've hit a "high" twice. But I could have been dehydrated. Or hormonal.

But I do it anyway. And I love that I do it. I love the fact that when I'm finished, I can check it off my list for that day or that week. That's my goal, just to do it—not to love it or to even like it while I'm doing it. I have found some things I do like or even love. I love bike riding, kickboxing, and rowing. But these are things I can't do very often because of the logistics of my life. So there's always running for me, and I've found ways to tolerate it while I'm on the trail or in the streets. If I expected every outing to give me some kind of high, I'd be constantly disappointed, and disappointment is one of the enemies of every would-be Former Fat Girl.

Designate a two-week trial period on your calendar.

Even though you might not fall in love with exercise—although that would be a pleasant surprise, wouldn't it?—there's some kind of workout out there that you will like enough to do several times a week. If, for instance, you don't already know that the stationary bike is more boring than school board meetings on local cable, the two-week trial period is the time to find out. The drill: Try at least two different fitness experiences— different cardio machines or classes at the health club; a variety of workout tapes; activities like swimming, walking, running, and cycling. Consider this a fact-finding mission. Which was the least objectionable? Is it tolerable enough and convenient enough for you to do several times a week?

Take more time if you need to, but it's better to put a deadline on this kind of thing. Otherwise, you could experiment forever and never commit—kind of like some guys I know.

Pick and stick.

At the end of the period, pick the activity that will work best for you and make a commitment to stick with it for at least six weeks. Why six weeks? That's the length of time researchers say it takes to build a habit. I don't know about that. If everything I ever did consistently for six weeks became a habit, I'd be a checkout girl at Kmart, eating popcorn every night for dinner, and wearing a royal blue LaCoste polo that a boy gave me in the eleventh grade. (I had a crush on him and refused to take it off.)

The six-week thing isn't set in stone, but you'll be doing great to get there. Once you do, technically you should be ready to work harder. Start using that 10 percent rule I explained above and see how you feel. I know that when I was starting out, any deviation from my routine—Jazzercise Monday, Wednesday, and Friday—threatened to suck me back into the Fat Girl lifestyle. If after the six weeks you feel the least bit precarious, stick with your original program.

Feel free to ignore the fitness experts who suggest switching your type of exercise to keep from getting bored and injured. Not that I want you to be bored or injured. Certainly, if you start feeling symptoms of either, get help. In the case of boredom, that might mean making your workout more challenging or trying something completely new for another six-

Kinder, Gentler Ways to Get Moving

To help you ease your way into exercise, here's a key to what's low impact, medium impact, and high impact, and the pros and cons of each.

Low Impact		
Activities	Pros	Cons
Swimming and water aerobics	Easy on your joints No sweat involved Total-body toning	The swimsuit issue Chlorine
Cycling	Great for butt and thighs Allows you to read (stationary bikes only, please!)	No upper-body involvement
Rowing	Major calorie-scorcher Total-body toning	Proper technique is tricky Machines in gyms are often rusty due to lack of use
Yoga, Pilates, Tai Chi	Combination of stretching, strengthening, and stress relief Little sweat Little equipment necessary	No cardio Need some instruction to get the most out of them
Strength training	Total-body toning (depending on program) Quick results (in upper body) Builds bone mass	Proper form is tricky Some risk of injury (due to improper form and lifting too much weight)

Medium Impact

Activities	Pros	Cons
Walking	Can do it anywhere, anytime Little equipment necessary Good total-body exercise if you swing your arms	Easy to get too comfortable with pace Can be hard on feet Can get boring
Stair climbers	Slims hips, thighs, and butt Can read while you work out	Can aggravate knee problems Easy to cheat by leaning on console
Elliptical trainers	Slims hips, thighs, and butt Can read while you work out	Easy to cheat by leaning on console Pushing/pulling arm handles can aggravate lower back problems
Aerobics and dance classes (no jumping)	Music and instructor can keep you motivated Total-body toning (depending on class) Includes warm-up, cool-down, and stretching to help prevent injury	Music and instructor can be annoying Requires coordination to execute steps Have to be able to fit into your schedule

High Impact

Activities	Pros	Cons
Running	Major calorie-scorcher Great self-esteem booster Little equipment necessary	Can be hard on feet and joints Overuse injuries common Can get boring
Kickboxing	Calorie scorcher Total-body toning Great for self-esteem (makes you feel tough!)	Proper technique is tricky Injuries common due to jumping and kicking
Aerobics and dance classes (jumping included)	Total-body toning High fun factor Music and instructor can keep you motivated	Injuries common due to jumping Requires coordination to execute steps Have to be able to fit into your schedule

week trial. On the injury front, stop what you're doing and call your doctor. In fact, that's a good thing for any beginner to do before starting an exercise program, especially if you've had health problems or some other reason for concern.

Use the sitcom strategy.

Somehow a thirty-minute workout seems more doable when you realize you're talking about the time it takes to watch a *Will & Grace* rerun (with commercials and credits). What's half an hour in the scheme of things? Nothing—except an opportunity to change your whole life.

Eat a taco.

My taco and ice cream workout chaser probably wouldn't be sanctioned by Weight Watchers, but it was a way of rewarding myself for doing something really, really hard and really, really out of character. I'm convinced I needed a reward to keep me going, like I used to reward my dog Yogi for resisting the innate urge to lunge for every squirrel with me in tow on the other end of the leash.

That's exactly what you are trying to do: resist your innate urges and train yourself to behave in a way that doesn't come naturally. So reward yourself once a day for the hard work you're doing. You deserve it. Plus, treating yourself will help keep you in "I can" mode. And it doesn't have to be with food; try a great manicure/pedicure, an hour all to yourself reading at the coffee shop, or the latest chick flick with your girlfriends.

And that's the magic of Secret #1: It helps you lay the can-do groundwork that will shore you up for the challenges of the journey ahead. If you can do this, if you can become the type of person for whom exercise is a habit (and I know you can), you have half the Former Fat Girl journey nailed. I know that without the juice I got from running, I never would have been able to make the transformation. The self-esteem boost, the changes I felt going on inside, spurred me on. Oh, and then there were the calories I was burning with every step.

But as you know, you don't do all this in a vacuum. Secret #2 will help you take on one of the toughest challenges of trying to lose weight in the real world in a way that most diets ignore: the influences of the people around you who unwittingly can keep you stuck where you are. Learning how to stay true to your plan amid all the advice and criticisms meant to be helpful but often anything but, will take you one step closer to making your Former Fat Girl dream a reality.

Chapter Two

Secret #2: Keep It a Secret

I remember the exact moment self-consciousness set in. I was about six years old, practicing for my first tap dance recital in an itchy, yolk-yellow tutu, my poor, bare little thighs jiggling as I shuffled. This was before parents shuttled their kids to a different activity every day of the week. Dance for me and Little League for my brothers—that was it. With four of us (my sister came along later), that was all the chauffering my parents could handle.

I don't recall too much about the classes themselves, which means they must not have been horrible. But I do remember the nervous anticipation building in the pit of my stomach as the recital approached. It was a big deal, probably the biggest deal up to that point in my young life: We were to perform on a stage, with a curtain and everything—just like the people on

Lawrence Welk, which my brothers and I were forced to watch with Mom and Dad on Saturday nights. I was so excited at the prospect of my star turn that I decided to give a sneak peek of my performance for the family, a decision I would soon regret.

We gathered in the living room of our house in suburban Boston. The relatively bright space with stiff, brocaded furniture and a light sprinkling of fragile knickknacks was typically off-limits to us kids. With the exception of holiday family photos, the living room was adult territory. We spent most of our family time in the basement den where there was a couch comfortable enough to actually sit on and, more important, where the only television we owned was situated.

Every so often my parents would set up card tables in our living room and have friends over to play poker or bridge. I loved it when they entertained, because the next morning I'd sneak down and pick through the scraps on the trays of leftover hors d'oeuvres. Sometimes Mom would leave the nut bowls out when she was too tired at the end of the night to clean up, and I'd scavenge for bits of cashew among the rejected Brazil nuts (which even *I* wasn't desperate enough to eat, at least most of the time).

So when Mom and Dad suggested we hold my private family performance in the living room, I was ecstatic. (Never mind that it was the only room in the house with a stereo, and it had a wood floor that was perfect for tapping.)

Mom and Dad corralled my three brothers into the straight-backed chairs we had set up for the "audience" as I stood on the hardwood floor "stage" in front of them, ready to do my thing. Someone—Dad, probably—introduced me and cued up the music. (I think it was our recital piece, the "Theme from the Pink Panther," but I'm not completely sure.) I started tapping away, searching for the rhythm, tentative at first, my confidence growing with each tap-tap-shuffle-ball-change. I even started showing off a bit, allowing myself to revel in the attention, sinking into it like a steamy bath on a frigid afternoon, and letting it wash over me.

You'd think I was used to all that attention, being the only girl in the family until my sister came along when I was eight. Not me. I defied the prima-donna, center-of-the-universe stereotype usually ascribed to only-girls. For one thing, I was somewhat of an introvert, so I kind of naturally receded into the background, spending hours reading and creating imaginary worlds in my head. Plus, I was a textbook example of the middle child. I had two older brothers: Henry, the buttoned-up, emotionally distant intellectual; Pete, the mischievous renegade (some would say troublemaker). Charlie, two years younger, was the loving baby (at least to my mom; he would prove to be my antagonist as he got older). Sandwiched in the middle was me—the peacekeeper, the pleaser, the good girl, the one who didn't want to make any waves. I craved my parents' approval, but I was uncomfortable being singled out for any reason, good *or* bad.

For instance, from a very young age I loved the fact that the family often celebrated my birthday and Pete's on the same day. Pete was two years and two days older than me, and our birthdays often ended up on top of the Thanksgiving holiday (mine is November 25, and Pete's is the 27th). Who could blame my mom for wanting to double up? When other kids would balk at sharing anything on their birthdays, especially attention, I was happy to make room for Pete. And he was—is—a natural ham, so he did a great job of creating a diversion.

Although I was comfortable with my place in the periphery, I must have had at least a little desire to step onto center stage. Why else would I be so ready to share my tap dancing talents with my family, especially my brothers, who I knew would be a tough crowd? I had been stung by their teasing before, so I knew what they were capable of. Still, I was willing to take the risk. Actually, I wasn't really aware of how much of a risk I was taking. See, while I might have had the beginnings of a Fat Girl body, I didn't have the Fat Girl psyche yet. Even though I didn't actively seek the spotlight, I wasn't yet fearful of it, fearful enough to hide from it at any cost.

That would all change.

There I was in my tutu, my stubby feet shuffling to the beat as best I could, all eyes on me. I was prancing, bathing in the limelight, completely ignorant of any imperfections in my step and oblivious to the way I looked as I bobbed along. My parents watched, encouraging, approving. I made it a point to avoid glancing in my brothers' direction; I knew they'd do anything—stick their tongues out, thumb their noses, moon me—to make me mess up.

As it turned out, I didn't need them to sabotage my performance. I took care of that by myself. All of a sudden, right before the big finish, it happened: My black patent Mary Janes slipped out from under me on the slick floor, and I fell—*smack*—right on my butt. I sat there a minute, too stunned to cry. I could feel my face burning with shame. My brothers dissolved into laughter, unable to restrain themselves. And who could blame them? This was almost as good as a front-row seat at a Three Stooges show.

My mother lunged to help me up. I pushed her away angrily and struggled to my feet. Dad was yelling at my brothers to shut up as I ran to my room, tears filling my eyes.

There I was, full of myself, performing, putting myself out

there (even if it was just for my family). I had allowed myself to shine like never before, and what did I get for it? I ended up on my ass and in tears, the butt of a family joke for years to come.

From then on, the last thing I wanted was to be in the spotlight. I wasn't safe there. I didn't know how to laugh it off. I didn't have the strength to set my jaw, dust off my bruised backside, and try again. Why risk that kind of pain when you can stay in the shadows, on the sidelines, a comfortable, content nobody?

Oh, I suffered through the class recital, of course. I was too much of a good girl to make a stink and quit. During the performance, I shrunk back into the second row, tapping very tentatively, too afraid to let myself go and enjoy the moment. Once the dance ordeal was over, I receded further into my imagination, into my books, into my own little world. As young as I was, I knew exactly what I was doing. No way was I going to give my brothers, my family—*anybody*—a reason to laugh at me. I'd show them. I would *disappear.*

It's not like I ever ran away or anything (that's not a good-girl thing, either), but I began disappearing, hiding, emotionally and physically. I simply stopped trying. I stopped trying to be heard in a household of constant noise and interruption. I stifled my interest in any kind of after-school activities. I abandoned any effort to pull myself out of my comfort zone, the safety of my own inner world.

Only part of my motive was self-preservation. The other part was the childish hope that someone would see my pain and rescue me from it. Like the runaway who secretly wishes for her parents to come after her, I yearned for mine to recognize my silent protest. I was trying to make a point, to let my family know (my parents in particular) how much the ridicule hurt me, to shame *them* for shaming *me*.

I actually devised a test for the family, a little game of hide-and-seek. I was the hider; they were the seekers. But here's the trick: They didn't know they were playing. They were supposed to notice my absence and become concerned enough to come looking for me. The problem was that no one ever did. I'd hole up behind one of the burnt orange and gold chairs in the forbidden living room, waiting to hear, "Has anybody seen Lisa? Where could she be?" Instead, the household clicked along without me, never noticing my absence. I'd give it about an hour—which seemed like forever—and then I'd resurface, going back to my books or my Barbies as if nothing had happened, all the while aching inside.

Sad, wasn't it? And I'm just getting started.

I struggled to conceal my emotions, afraid of being teased and laughed at. Crying was a big no-no. I remember when the movie *Brian's Song* was on TV for the first time—the story of the pro football player who dies of leukemia after standing up for his friendship with an African American player. A classic tearjerker. Watching the movie in the den with my family, I moved from the couch to the floor as the plot became more and more upsetting. I lay on my stomach with my hands cupped around my face so no one would see my tears. I used that strategy while viewing many a made-for-TV movie over the years.

And God forbid that anyone—my brothers or my Dad, especially—suspected me of having a crush on a *boy*. They'd launch into a rendition of "Lisa and [boy's name here] sitting in a tree, k-i-s-s-i-n-g," or torture me with smooching noises on the rare occasion that a boy actually called me on the phone. In response, I learned to hide those feelings, too. I was embarrassed by them, almost as embarrassed as I was when I slipped and fell that day in the living room.

As I shut out the outside world, my inner world exploded with life. I daydreamed constantly, conjuring up entire relationships and conversations with kids at school or in the neighborhood—kids I didn't have the nerve to speak to. I lived through my books, diving into the worlds created by the authors. I loved books by Judy Blume whose heroines were often girls like me, girls on the outside looking in. I loved Nancy Drew, because she was so *not* like me—taking chances, speaking up, stepping forward. I loved Jo in *Little Women*. I wanted to *be* her, the instigator, the driven one, the champion of self-expression. I read whatever I could get my hands on, and when I found a favorite, I went back to it repeatedly, revisiting the characters as if they were old friends.

When I was in fifth or sixth grade, I discovered *Harriet the Spy* by Louise Fitzhugh. Harriet was this little mousy kid, kind of nerdy and supersmart, the underdog protagonist typical of many books for preteens and teens. (Think Hermione from the Harry Potter series, without the wand.) Harriet fashioned herself as some kind of secret agent, keeping notes on the kids and goings-on around her.

Like me, Harriet had a secret life, a life where she could be smarter, more creative, stronger, braver. Where she could be everything she wanted to be—everything she felt she couldn't be in the real world.

No wonder I related.

I was hardly the only kid who was ever teased or experienced some kind of spectacular failure. There are millions of them: the directionally challenged peewee football player who scores a touchdown for the other team; the unfortunate girl who is caught without a pad when she starts her period and everyone can tell (by the way, that happened to me, too); the stomach virus victim who pukes on her desk during second period (uh, me again). There are certainly worse things that can happen to children, that *do* happen to children. All you have to do is watch one of those twenty-four-hour news channels to know your place in this sad spectrum. The blooper reel of my childhood is nothing compared to what some people— maybe even you—have gone through.

I don't blame my parents for not protecting me or my brothers for, well, being brothers. But for some reason, comments that might have rolled off other kids penetrated my spirit like needles in a cushion. You know how it feels when every slight stings like a slap, every joke belies a secret truth, every criticism is a condemnation. And any mistake I made, however minor, only served to support my sneaking suspicion: *I am worthless.*

In response, I shut down. I activated a defense mechanism that I used for many, many years to safeguard the vulnerable parts of myself from outside scrutiny. And part of that defense was my weight.

As I grew older and heavier, my weight became a way of hiding. It gave me an excuse to retreat from tryouts for school plays, from band and choir and sports. Not only that, the weight itself became a cloak, like the cloak Harry Potter and his pals throw on when they want to make themselves invisible. That is exactly how I began to feel, how I wanted to feel: invisible.

I continued to pile on the pounds, stuffing myself as covertly as possible to avoid having to deal with my mother's sympathy or my brothers' ridicule (both were equally annoying). I became a master at hiding, sneaking, and stashing food. If there was a can of frosting in the fridge, my finger had been in it. Chocolate syrup? I'd take a swig from the can while no one was looking. Cookie crumbs in my pockets, candy wrappers in my closet—it's a wonder we didn't have a mouse problem. I was like one of those cartoonish portrayals of an alcoholic who has bottles stashed everywhere—in the toilet tank, under the piano lid, inside a hollowed-out book.

I did all the family baking, not because I was "Mommy's little helper" but because I knew that inevitably a smidgen of dough or a dribble of batter would find its way into my mouth. And once the goodies were out of the oven, I'd use my sneaky skills to nibble away at them without anyone noticing (or so I thought). A sheet cake with a couple of pieces missing was an easy target. I'd find my way into the kitchen while everyone else was occupied and start trimming away at it. I'd never cut myself an actual piece—just a sliver here, a sliver there to "even out the row." In the process, I'd end up eating half the pan. It was kind of like when you start plucking your eyebrows just to clean them up, and by the time you're finished, you look like one of those hairless cats fancied by people with allergies (and some New York socialites).

With every covert kitchen operation, my stockpile of shame grew larger. I was so ashamed of what I was doing, but I couldn't stop myself. You know how it is: You promise yourself never again. This is the last time, the last bite. And then your hand is back in the cookie jar again. *Just one more.* Shame is a powerful thing, but it's no match for the appetite of a Fat Girl.

Of course, everyone knew what I was doing. It was as obvious as my growing belly, butt, and thighs (not to mention the chocolate under my fingernails). I was the only one in the house who would even consider sneaking food. If my brothers wanted to eat something, they just went ahead and did it. They didn't skulk around in shame, afraid to acknowledge their appetite, humiliated by their lack of self-control. I had the corner on that market.

Little did I know that all that secretiveness would become one of the keys to becoming a Former Fat Girl. Here's how it happened.

Every so often, starting probably around the fifth or sixth grade, I'd go on a diet. Maybe there was a boy who caught my eye, or maybe I caught sight of my increasingly chunky body at just the right (wrong?) angle in the mirror, or maybe it was getting to be more of a struggle than usual to button my pants. Whatever it was, something inspired me to stop the pounds from piling on.

At that time, "going on a diet" to me meant skipping dessert or snacking on celery instead of chips or stopping just short of eating until it hurt on the rare occasions that the family went out to dinner. Back then, in the early 70s, ten-year-old girls simply weren't sophisticated enough about the whole subject of dieting to know the ins and outs of plans like Atkins or Weight Watchers. Not like today when girls learn to live in fear of carbs and fat grams before they get their first training bra.

Of course, our moms knew the score. That was when Atkins first hit the scene, when even the toniest restaurant offered the diet plate (a bunless hamburger patty, cottage cheese, and cling peaches), and amphetamines were the drugs of choice for weight-conscious models and suburban moms. Not my mom. Despite the fact that she and I shared the same pear shape, I don't remember her being into any of that. But a woman whose four kids I used to babysit was always doing something to try to lose her postpartum pounds. In her pantry she kept a box of a "diet candy" with the unfortunate name of Aids. (I found it one night when I was foraging for snacks after the kids went to sleep—one of the Fat Girl perks for babysitting.) It was so named because they "aided" women who were trying to lose weight. Aids were half-inch, chocolate- or vanilla-flavored cubes almost as chewy as Tootsie Rolls but not nearly as tasty. I am sure they contained caffeine, at the very least, or maybe some now illegal appetite suppressant. The things never did much for me, but then I don't think they were meant to be taken as a chaser after a junk food binge, in the desperate hope that they would somehow undo the damage.

At the time I didn't realize what a mistake it was to "announce" that I was dieting. I wanted my family—Mom and Dad, especially—to know that I was trying. I could see how relieved and happy they were when I courageously passed up a second helping or a dish of the chocolate pudding Mom often made for dessert. I made a big show of it, feeding their expectations, winning their approval. After all, they desperately wanted to help me; they hated to see me miserable, lonely, and stuffing myself.

And that actually turned out to be the problem. By going public with my diet, I basically invited everyone in my family to "help." Now they could voice, in the spirit of helping, all those hints, tips, and wise observations they had been keeping to themselves. They had free rein to police my plate, to point out any breach of the rules I had so publicly proclaimed. They didn't have to hold back: They could remind me how fattening mashed potatoes are and that Oreos aren't exactly diet food and that between-meal snacking really puts on the pounds. As if I didn't know.

"Are you *sure* you want that?" "Is that on your diet?" These were innocent questions, I know, posed with the best of intentions, but to me they sounded like stinging criticisms, expressions of doubt and distrust. I heard "You aren't strong enough to lose the weight on your own. You can't be trusted to make your own decisions about how to manage your appetite. You're a wimp."

All those questions and comments simply confirmed what I already believed deep inside: I was weak. I couldn't do it. And they made me want to shove away the diet plate, tuck into the all-you-can-eat platter, and give up altogether.

My brothers only made things worse. They used my diet proclamation to push my buttons. "Some diet *that* is!" one might say when I put something decidedly undietlike on my plate. Or "*Mom*, is Lisa allowed to have a cookie?" Not quite the supportive atmosphere you need when you're trying to break a hardwired overeating habit.

To my parents I'd mumble something like "No, I guess I *don't* need a handful of chips while I watch the *Flintstones*." To my brothers I'd react with a shrewish "Shut up!"—all the while planning a secret rendezvous with the snack jar the first chance I got.

When it was obvious that their help wasn't exactly helping, my parents held back their comments as best they could and tried to get my brothers to stifle theirs. But the damage was done. After the first or second time I "came out" as a dieter, I figured out just how alert the family became to every spoonful I put on my plate, every forkful that made it to my mouth. Their comments echoed in my mind as real as if they were repeated out loud. If I had any notion that telling them would help me keep my promise to myself, the reality was just the opposite: All it took was one look, a raised eyebrow, the flash of a frown, and my resolve to lose the weight would crumble. I'd go right back to sneaking food every chance I got.

The worst thing was that every time I failed to keep my

vow to lose weight, I disappointed not only myself but my parents. To me, people-pleasing middle child me, that made my failure all the more devastating. I had gotten everyone's hopes up, not just mine, and then shot them right back down. Why put all of us through it again?

That was my thinking when, years later, I finally started my journey to becoming a Former Fat Girl. I made a conscious decision not to tell anyone—neither my family nor my friends—about going to Jazzercise. After all, I would have to describe to them exactly what Jazzercise was, and I could imagine the visions they would conjure up. The fact that I was exercising at all would seem strange enough, let alone frolicking around in tights with my legs looking like bratwurst bulging out of its casings.

The only one who knew was Tracey, who got me hooked on the class in the first place. Tracey understood the whole Fat Girl thing because she was one, too. She knew what it was like to feel that someone was constantly monitoring you, just waiting for you to screw up. It was an unwritten, unspoken vow between us: I won't play that game if you won't.

I was living in Austin, and my parents were two and a half hours away by car in Houston, so it wasn't as if I had to sneak around for fear of being caught or anything. Even so, it was a struggle for me not to say anything, especially after I became a regular at Jazzercise. For one thing, I was excited about this new development in my life. I was discovering a part of myself, a seed of confidence, that I never knew was there. I wanted to gush about it to someone and even brag a bit. I yearned to see my parents' faces light up with that hope, that pride, that approval I knew they would feel at the idea that I was again trying to wrench myself out of that unhappy, unhealthy place I had been in for so long.

But I held back from them, from my brothers, and from my other friends. It was hard to hide for too long, of course. As I started to lose weight, it became obvious that I was doing something differently. Even so, I said very little. If anyone asked, I responded in the most nonchalant, off-the-cuff kind of way: "Oh, I've been going to some exercise class," as if it were the most normal thing in the world when it was anything but. It was like saying you were "just going shopping" when you were really jetting off to Paris for the fall fashion shows.

I simply didn't trust myself to stick with it, to follow through. After all, I had never followed through in the past. Then when I started running, I became even more secretive. Running seemed so much more athletic and out of reach for a Fat Girl like me. I was no Olympian; who was I to think I could run? Not only did I go to the track under the cover of dark (note: not recommended for safety reasons; I never said I was smart about it), but I ran alone. For a very long time—long after I had started running every day, five miles a day, on the trail around Lake Austin that "real" runners frequent—I refused to run with anyone else. Frankly, I was afraid I'd be too slow or look too stupid. I was afraid of being judged and not measuring up. That sounds crazy, right? After all, other runners who happened to be on the trail at the time could see how fast or slow I was going, how goofy I looked in my shorts and tights. (Yes, I wore tights under my running shorts for years, afraid to let loose my thighs.)

It's funny, though. The strangers I could deal with. Somehow I talked myself into the idea that if I didn't make eye contact with the other runners passing me on the trail, I would be invisible to them. Looking them in the eye let them into my world, into my head, where they could pull up a chair, sit down, and proceed to destroy my budding confidence by tick-ing off all the reasons I didn't belong there. Averting my gaze sealed off that tiny sprout of self-esteem like a vault, protecting it so it could continue to grow.

Friends were a different story. If Tracey had been at all interested in running, I probably would have let her come with me. I trusted her more than anyone I knew at the time because of her status as a Fat Girl and the nonjudgmental way she was with me. Even so, what if she ran faster than me? I'd feel like a loser, like I did in junior high when I was always picked last (or next to last) by the team captains in gym class. Or what if she was slower? That would be almost as bad. I might have to use on her some of the mental energy I devoted to getting myself through the run. And I had none to spare.

No, I had to do it alone. I had to do it at my pace, in my way, with no one to compare myself to or to compete with. I didn't know it then, but I was really giving myself time and space to make exercise a habit. I was laying a foundation, allowing the cement to dry thoroughly before testing it.

The food thing was harder. People are always so curious about what other people are eating. Have you ever noticed how in restaurants people crane their necks to see what the waiter is bringing out? The contents of your dinner plate are, I submit, even more snoop-worthy than what's in your medicine cabinet. It's even worse when you're a guest in someone's house. The cook is always checking what you're eating and how much—she measures the success of the meal by the size of portions, the number of helpings, and the quantities of leftovers on plates and in bowls. She notes the disposition of every morsel, doing a kind of mental calculus, urging her guests to eat more to tip the balance in her favor.

Normal people are food-focused in normal situations.

Throw a dieting Fat Girl into the mix, and everyone is on high alert. In that case, it's not just the hostess doing the tabulating. All those who know your situation are, even if they're not boorish enough to say anything.

Solitary confinement at mealtime isn't the only way to get around this, but it's not such a bad idea if you can swing it, at least at first. Once I started my Former Fat Girl journey, I took a hiatus from going out with friends to eat (or drink, because we'd usually end up eating, too) for at least two months. I was living alone at the time, so in effect I ate solo at just about every meal for a while. I didn't have to deal with the prying eyes of my fellow diners. I didn't have to deal with the temptation posed by a companion's big, greasy bacon cheeseburger or platter of spaghetti when all I had was a bowl of greens, dressing on the side.

When I did start venturing out again, I tried to keep my dietary restrictions as inconspicuous as possible. Ordering at restaurants was tough; I did ask whether the chicken was fried or grilled and requested vegetables without butter. But I always tried to have a quick default option so that I wouldn't have to get into a lengthy negotiation with the waiter. (You know that tedious litany of questions and qualifications: Can I have the fish? Make it grilled, not fried, in just a drop or two of oil, not butter. I would like the side of vegetables that comes with the tenderloin, but not the cream sauce; maybe just a drop or two of vinaigrette.) Salad was my fallback solution. I choked down a lot of it in those days.

I could hardly demand to have a special meal prepared at people's homes or in cases when there was a set menu (at a business dinner, for instance). In those circumstances I would just deal with it. If the food was already plated, I'd eat what I could and push around the other stuff; if we were helping ourselves, I'd take a larger portion of acceptable foods—veggies, salad, chicken or fish—and small bits of the other stuff. I learned to put at least a bite of everything on my plate to avoid raising questions from the cook: "Oh, don't you like macaroni and cheese? Mine is an old family recipe. Here, let me give you enough to feed a family of four." I often left the stuff untouched, but at the end of the meal my plate would look no different from the plates of others who started out with five times that amount.

I know what you're thinking: How could you *not* eat what's on your plate? Fat Girls don't leave food on their plate unless it's truly inedible, and even then we have to take several bites to make sure. This shows you the power of Secret #1. Through exercise I had begun to build the strength and stamina to say no to my appetite, to put down the fork before my plate was clean. After all, every time I hit that track I was doing something I thought was impossible. If I could run three laps, a mile, two miles, maybe I could leave that last bite on the plate.

But Secret #2: Keep It a Secret is just as important. It will help you insulate yourself from the doubts, criticism, and "helpful" input that could sidetrack you as you work the Former Fat Girl program. Without Secret #2, your whole future as a Former Fat Girl is at risk. Read on to see how you can make it work for you.

Fly Below the Radar

Weight loss gurus usually tell you to share your goals to make you feel accountable to someone else and to garner support for the task you're undertaking. Their reason is that if everyone, or at least someone, knows you're dieting, you're less likely to

cheat. Maybe that's true for some people, but for future Former Fat Girls, I say that's risky business.

I know what it's like to feel as if someone is monitoring
every bite you take or, worse, nagging you outright to exercise. It's hard not to get resentful; it's hard not to take every
helpful suggestion and innocent question as a criticism or ac-
cusation, as a reminder that you're too weak to do it on your
own—or even that you can't do it at all. Instead of keeping
you from "cheating," it drives you underground where you
indulge in secret. That only feeds the burning shame inside you.

I mean, how many times did I use the "I'm on a diet" excuse for ordering a skimpy dressing-on-the-side salad for dinner, only to turn around the next day, the next week, or the
next month and polish off an entire plate of fettuccine Alfredo?
Who would blame a well-meaning spouse or friend for asking,
"Are you *supposed* to be eating that?" And who would blame
you for being offended? It's enough to make you want to order
a second dessert out of spite.

That's why it's better to stay under the radar. Don't make
a big deal about the fact that you're exercising; just do it. As
foreign as it might feel to you, try to act as if it's the most natural thing in the world, like going to the grocery store or taking
your clothes to the cleaners. Don't announce at the dinner table "I'm on a diet" when you order a grilled chicken breast instead of a burger and fries. You don't have to explain yourself.
You just happen to be in the mood for chicken.

Keeping your quest for your new life a secret will help insulate you from the scrutiny and expectations of others. I've
found (after lots of fits and starts) that if you don't make a big deal
of it, other people will be more likely to follow your lead.

It will be tempting to share with the people around you

that you really are going to do something about your weight, that this time will be different. You think that if they know you're trying, they'll be a little less judgmental, a little less critical, a little less likely to write you off as "just a Fat Girl"—not the unique, wonderfully talented, truly compassionate, insightful woman you are. You think it will make the people you love happy, because you know they have been suffering with you, too. You think it will stop the teasing, the nagging, the outright insults—spoken and unspoken.

It will also be tempting to share because you need support, you need coaching, and you need cheerleading. You're doing something extraordinary, something that few people are able to do or even willing to try. You are entering a period of rebirth, attempting to shed the thought patterns and behaviors that have come to define who you are. You are assuming a new identity, like a mobster who turns against the boss and goes into the witness protection program—except that you don't have the FBI to create a new life for you; you have to do it yourself. (Hmmm. I've been watching too much *Law & Order*. But you get the picture.)

Well, here's the thing: There are ways to get the emotional stuff you need while protecting yourself from the outside influences that could drag you down. And here's another upside of keeping your secret: You'll begin to learn to rely on your own inner reserve to keep you motivated, to give you willpower. You may ask: *What* reserve? *What* willpower? Believe me, it's there. It just hasn't had a good workout in a while. Willpower is like a muscle; it can only grow and strengthen if you use it. As you reduce your dependency on others for motivation and begin to focus inward, you'll be surprised at how strong you really are.

Now, let's get to it: How do you change your life without

your husband/significant other/nosy roommate finding out? What do you do if you're struggling and really need support? My Former Fat Girl fixes will help you deal with these challenges and more.

The Obstacle: Well-Meaning but Nosy People Who Want to Help

Unless you're a hermit, it's really tough to turn your life around completely without anyone noticing. Even so, there are ways to protect your secret or at least keep from attracting so much attention that it undermines everything you're trying to do.

Former Fat Girl Fixes

Be a little antisocial.

Try to sequester yourself as much as possible, especially when you first begin your journey to Former Fat Girlhood. Avoid going out to eat or at least set a strict limit (once a week or even less often). Exercise solo (if you can stand it), and if you're trying a fitness class or going to a gym, avoid busy hours and try not to attend a class with people you know. Why the loner act? Think about this. You might be doing all you can to change, but the people around you still see you as the person you have been all along. Just being around familiar people and in familiar situations can force you back into the very thought and behavior patterns you're trying to break. I am not making this up: Drug and alcohol recovery programs often cut addicts off from family and friends for a period of time to help them wipe the slate clean and, in effect, start their lives over. The addict's situation is more extreme, of course, but when you think about it, there are a lot of parallels between what you're trying to do and what a recovering addict tries to do. You are shedding the image you've had of yourself for years—maybe all your life. You are learning how to act differently and think differently. You're trying to find new sources of fun and pleasure that don't revolve around food. You may be evolving into a new you, but your family and friends still think of you as the Fat Girl they know and love. You need space and time for your new habits to take hold so that you won't fall back into that old Fat Girl role.

I was lucky that I lived alone at the time of my Fat Girl to Former Fat Girl conversion. I decided what to keep in my pantry and fridge because I didn't have other non-wannabe Former Fat Girls to accommodate. I could get away with eating a light dinner. I didn't have to deal with kids who need Cheetos for their lunch boxes and want macaroni and cheese for dinner every night or a husband with a fetish for ice cream. That's what trips you up. It's too easy to slip a handful of Cheetos into your mouth when you're packing lunches and to polish off the leftover macaroni in the kitchen during cleanup. (Stay tuned for Secret #3. It will help you battle the urge to indulge and sneak.)

Keep it brief.

What you do with your life is your business. It's easy to feel that you need to offer information about your new exercise routine or your diet plan, but the truth is, you don't. Only allude to your journey if someone comments, and even in that case, avoid lengthy explanations. Just say in the most offhand, casual way that you went for a walk or you had a salad for dinner or whatever. Don't get into the whole "I'm going to change my life once and for all" thing. Just respond in as few words as possible and change the subject.

I'm not telling you to turn into an uncommunicative jerk. You should definitely use your better judgment so that you don't offend someone with your terseness. But recognize this: When you're a Fat Girl, you are wrapped up in your struggles with food, with your appetite, and with your body in ways that other people aren't. As curious as they might be about what other people order in a restaurant or whether their dinner guests really like the spinach soufflé, others don't have a 24-7 tape in their heads blaring a litany of everything they have eaten and why they shouldn't have eaten it. (Don't you wonder sometimes what they do think about?)

They are simply not as tuned in to the whole food thing as you are, and they're certainly not preoccupied with or even all that interested in your entire history of dieting. They don't expect you to put this new effort you're making into context and to expound on why this approach is better than the last one. So don't go there. If you do, you might end up embroiled in a discussion that can lead to, for instance, a debate on your approach to dieting or how often you should work out or whatever. And all that will do is make you doubt yourself. You don't need any more self-doubt than you already have.

Issue a gag order.

I know you might feel uneasy at the idea of keeping something so important from the people closest to you. Secrecy could have serious consequences, after all. You don't want your husband to think you're working up a sweat at the Motel 6 when you're really trudging on the treadmill at the Y, for example.

But be careful when you break it to whoever you think really needs to know. Sit down with him face-to-face as if you're getting ready to have the most serious of conversations. Use whatever tone or body language you reserve for those heavy, deep, and real discussions so he knows you mean business. Tell him you're really determined this time and appreciate his concern and support. Ask him to let you bring up the subject when you want to talk about it. Assure him that you'll let him know how you're doing when you're ready. That might keep him from making comments and asking questions that he thinks are helpful and supportive but that you might hear as nagging or judgmental.

Remember, they mean well.

Despite all your best efforts, though, you will inevitably get into exactly the conversation you want to avoid, the one where you hear that so-and-so tried the diet you're on and *gained* thirty pounds; or that walking on the treadmill isn't enough—you *really* should lift weights, too; or that those meal-replacement bars you're eating have as many calories as half a turkey sandwich, so why don't you just eat one of those? You end up feeling as if you're doing this all wrong, that it's not going to happen, that it's too confusing to figure out, so why even try? But wait. Before you talk yourself out of this whole Former Fat Girl thing, remember: They are just trying to help. They are not out to sabotage you. They don't think you're weak. They have no idea how these kinds of "helpful" hints and suggestions affect you. Try to smile and nod, say thanks for the information, and ask them what's the first thing they would do if they were president or something equally as complicated. And if they persist in offering unsolicited and unwelcome advice, talk to them about it. Don't let it go on. You don't want anything to take your focus off your goals. Use the gag-order strategy outlined above, making sure to thank them for their advice and concern but letting them know you would prefer that they allow you to bring up the subject in the future. I know you are cringing at the idea that you would actually have to do this, but trust me: It's a great feeling to learn to speak your mind and confront such situations, and in most cases you'll get what you want out of it.

The Obstacle: How to Stay Motivated Without Anyone to Support You

I'm asking you to get some distance from the people you normally rely on when you're having trouble coping and need a lift. So where do you turn if you can't go to them? Here are some ideas.

Former Fat Girl Fixes

Use the Internet.

Keeping your process to yourself is integral to becoming a Former Fat Girl, but I know it's hard to take on such a challenge completely on your own. You need to be able to tap into a support system to get you through tough times, and online communities for weight loss and exercise devotees are perfect for that. They can give you an emotional boost while preserving your anonymity. If you have ever visited a chat room, you know cyber relationships can become as dysfunctional as face-to-face ones. But your cyber supporters only know what you

The Best Online Support Groups for Future Former Fat Girls

Thousands and maybe millions of dieters are chronicling their hopes, dreams, hits, and misses on the Internet. Good for them and good for you. Online support groups, blogs, and diet success sites can give you the motivation and inspiration you need while maintaining your anonymity. At the same time, though, you don't want to find yourself on a site that is dishing out bogus info or that is merely a shill for some kind of flaky or dangerous diet aid. I have scrolled through scads of sites to come up with the following list of URLs worth a double click.

- eDiets.com (www.ediets.com). This site offers great success stories (with before and after photos) and more than eighty different support groups. The site is run by a staff of doctors and nutritionists, so you can be pretty confident of its credibility. The only problem is, you have to pay about $2 a week. If you're cheap like me, you might want to try some of the other free services first.

- WebMD (www.webmd.com). Another class operation, WebMD offers four Dieting Club message boards: one for people who want to lose 10 to 25 pounds, one for 25- to 50-pound losers, another for 50- to 100-pound losers, and another for 100-plus losers. The boards are monitored, so there is no danger of potty talk. You will read about confessions ("I just ate 7 chocolate hearts!") and triumphs ("I did my first triathlon!") and have the chance to encourage and applaud just as others encourage and applaud you. Oh, and this one's free.

- National Weight Control Registry (www.nwcr.ws). This site was started by two weight loss researchers who wanted to learn from successful losers, people who have lost 30 pounds or more and kept it off for one year. The profiles on the site will truly get and keep you going.

- Our Lady of Weight Loss (www.ourladyofweightloss.com). Kitschy as all get-out but completely fun, this site was created by self-proclaimed "weight loss artist" Janice Taylor. Her weekly e-newsletter, The KICK in the TUSH Club, will remind you that you're not in this alone.

- Weight Watchers.com (www.weightwatchers.com). No, you don't have to be on the diet to post, but I have to put in a plug for WW because it is the plan that helped me get where I am today. (You'll read about that later.) Not only are there message boards categorized by weight loss goals, but there are different boards for moms, students, brides-to-be, and even vegetarians.

tell them. They are not around to see that your jeans aren't any looser than they were last week. They can't point at the wall clock and ask, "Isn't your Pilates class in two minutes? Why aren't you there?" Frankly, you don't even need to post anything yourself to get a lift from them. Just reading about what other group members are going through can underscore the fact that you're not in this alone. And you might even find yourself offering advice based on your experience, which can really boost your confidence (so maybe I'm not so bad at this after all!). You can find great communities through IVillage and WebMD and, of course, through my Web site, FormerFatGirl.com.

Get a trainer.

First things first: Personal trainers are not just for people who have zero body fat or perfect measurements or who someday aspire to the Olympics. Trainers work with all kinds, from the superfit athlete to the cardiac rehab patient. Even so, the idea of working out with a personal trainer might make you kind of nervous. But the trainers I know are like the best coaches and the least annoying cheerleaders rolled into one. If they know what your goals are, they can push you just enough so that every workout is challenging but successful. The trick is to find one you click with. (See the sidebar on page 70 for tips on finding a trainer you can trust.) You need someone with whom you're not embarrassed to talk about your goals and your challenges, because communication is extremely important. If you're too embarrassed to tell her that you haven't worked out in, like, *ever* or that there's an excruciating pain in your back when you try a particular exercise, you're not going to get the most out of your workout and might even get hurt.

Once you've found your match, a trainer can be indispensable in several ways. Her technical expertise in exercise (and nutrition, provided she has the credentials) is only part of it. She'll also be there for you when your motivation flags. And because you have a professional relationship, there's less of a chance you'll resent her when she calls you on missing a workout. You can always fire her; the same is not true of your mother.

Write it down.

Sometimes all you need is to vent. You don't need advice or encouragement. You just need to get it all out. Journaling allows you to blow off steam and even work through some issues without having to deal with backtalk from a second party. This is not an original idea: Many weight loss experts suggest keeping a journal along with a log of what you're eating and how much you're exercising. Not only will that help keep you "honest"—which you may need because you can't rely on the power of peer pressure—but it is a great way to chronicle your progress. Full disclosure: Journaling has never really been my thing. I've always thought I *should* journal (don't most real writers?), but I've never been able to keep it up. I've amassed an extensive collection of beautiful volumes that remain blank except for two or three pages. I did, though, keep track of my weekly weigh-ins on my office calendar when I went on Weight Watchers and for a long time after I had reached my goal weight. I also kept a food log as part of that program and jotted down the number of miles I ran each day. Paging through, seeing the pounds drop and the miles tick up, was such a powerful experience. It was a visual, tactile affirmation of all the work I'd been doing. The only thing better? Squeezing into a smaller jeans size.

Find another Fat Girl or, even better,
a Former Fat Girl.

I was lucky to have Tracey when I started my own journey to
Former Fat Girlhood. Not all fellow Fat Girls are as accepting
and compassionate as Tracey. There are those who will tear
you down so they can feel better about themselves (such as that
stupid Mary Ann in third grade). There are those who will try
to keep you from changing because they're afraid of changing
themselves. There are those who simply are fighting their own
battles and might take you down with them when they back-
slide. So latching onto another Fat Girl isn't a surefire solution.
Teaming up with a Former Fat Girl, though, is a much safer
tactic. We know exactly what you're going through; we know
what worked for us; and we know how to share just enough
information and then back off and leave you alone. The problem is, you can't recognize us when you see us. That is the
point of this book: to let you know we're out there waiting to
help and cheering you on. But here is a hint that will help you
start your search: Some of the women most dedicated to exercise are Former Fat Girls. Aerobic instructors, trainers, marathon runners, triathletes—I can guarantee that if you tap into
that network, you'll find a Former Fat Girl or two, or three, or
more.

The Obstacle: Sticky Social Situations That Involve Food

Work parties, family gatherings, and nights out with the girls
can't be avoided completely. You just need to be prepared to
cope. These fixes will help.

Former Fat Girl Fixes

Play offense.

Let's say you're invited to a backyard barbecue and the cook's specialty is baby back ribs, something you'd rather not touch for fear of losing all control and eating an entire rack. Barbecues are particularly challenging for the wannabe Former Fat Girl because the traditional menu isn't exactly what you'd call healthy: potato salad, coleslaw, and macaroni salad dripping in mayo; baked beans swimming with chunks of bacon; and marbled meats oozing with oily sauces. If you are lucky, you might be able to scrounge up a lean piece of beef brisket or strip a chicken breast of its skin, and maybe snag a piece of white bread, but that's about it.

There are a couple of ways to deal with this situation without calling unwanted attention to yourself. (Staying home is not an option.) Eat something before you go—not a full meal but a heavy snack—say, half a peanut butter or turkey sandwich or a small bowl of cereal or some tuna over mixed greens. Then *nibble* at the party. Don't skip the meal altogether (see the next fix to find out why); instead, take small tasting portions of the dishes on the menu. But that strategy will backfire completely if you do let go at the party and eat a full meal. Another way to handle it is to bring a healthy side dish to share, making sure you get a substantial portion and leaving just a little space on your plate for the host's dishes. That way you'll have something to enjoy along with everyone else. Plus, you'll earn points for your "thoughtful" contribution to the meal—even though your motivation was more self*ish* than self*less*.

How to Find a Trainer Who Will Nudge You, Not Judge You

There are three major reasons to hook up with a personal trainer: motivation, expertise, and accountability. But in your head there are probably just as many reasons not to, the main one being fear. With the right trainer, though, fear won't be a factor at all. Here's how to make the best match:

Certification. Find a trainer who is certified by one of the organizations on this list:

Aerobic and Fitness Association of America (AFAA)

American College of Sports Medicine (ACSM)

American Council on Exercise (ACE)

Cooper Institute for Aerobics Research (CIAR)

International Sports Sciences Association (ISSA)

National Academy of Sports Medicine (NASM)

National Council of Strength and Fitness (NCSF)

National Federation of Professional Trainers (NFPT)

National Strength and Conditioning Association (NSCA)

This ensures that she has been thoroughly tested in anatomy and physiology, nutrition, exercise prescription, and CPR training. There are many certification programs out there, but they aren't as rigor-ous. These are your best bets, according to the consumer watchdog Web site Quackwatch.com.

Focus on women only. Men are pitiful enough when it comes to relat-ing to women in general, but to a wannabe Former Fat Girl? No way. A male trainer is going to be so removed from the Fat Girl way of thinking that it is doubtful you would make much progress. There's probably an exception among the thousands of trainers out there, but you would lose a lot of time finding him.

Be cautious about lifelong athletes. For some people, being active just comes naturally—but not you (not yet, anyway). Trainers who grew up playing soccer, lacrosse, softball, whatever, will probably have a difficult time relating to you and your struggles. You want to have as much common ground with your trainer as possible so she can anticipate your emotional needs as much as your physical needs. There are exceptions here, too. Maybe the athlete had a battle with her weight at some point in her life or had a Fat Girl for a sister or close friend.

Look for a Former Fat Girl. Former Fat Girls are like people who have undergone a religious conversion: They're often driven to spread the gospel to others. There's a great chance that you can find a trainer who went through the whole Fat Girl thing herself and took up train-ing in her zeal to share her new life with others. As you know, though, you can't tell a Former Fat Girl by looking at her. But all you'll need is one short conversation to find out. If she is truly a Former Fat Girl, she won't be able to keep it to herself. On the off-chance that she doesn't volunteer the information, ask, "Has it always been easy for you to stay fit?" That will get her talking about her own history.

Avoid critics and know-it-alls. In your conversation, tell her what you've been doing to lose weight or strategies you used in the past. Listen carefully to her response. Does she say, "Well, that's not going to get you where you want to be," or does she say, "Are you making any progress?" with a knowing smile on her face? Even if she disagrees with the tactics you're using, she shouldn't jump all over them. She should gently say, "I can help you with that," or "There are other ways," or even "There may be a better way." You need to be handled gently and be applauded for trying. Her manner in this discussion will help reveal whether she'll do that for you.

Could she be a confidant? Years ago I had a yellow Lab named Yogi. All Yogi wanted to do was please me, even more than eating and fetching, which is saying a lot. And that was great except for when he did something wrong such as wet the rug or chew up the newspaper or get into the refrigerator and eat a week's worth of groceries. Then he would hide from me. He wanted to please me so much that he couldn't bear to disappoint; he couldn't own up to his mistakes.

What does my dog have to do with you? Well, lots of trainer-client relationships are like my relationship with Yogi. The client—you—want so much to please that if you screw up, if you stray from your diet or don't do your weekend walks or whatever, you just can't face the trainer and end up severing the relationship out of guilt. As you talk to a potential trainer, ask yourself: What happens—worst-case scenario— if I slack off? Could I tell her? Would I come right back again, share my struggle, and move on? Or would I abandon the program altogether?

Don't refuse food.

This was a particularly hard lesson for me to learn. It would make sense that if you don't want to eat something, you shouldn't put any on your plate, right? Unfortunately, it doesn't work that way. Think about it: What would happen if you passed up a serving of your mom's special family recipe cheesecake with a simple "No, thank you"? If you think you'd get away with that, you've got another think coming. In my house, I'd be subjected to such interrogation and commentary, you'd think I was the latest nominee to the Supreme Court. It's better to accept some and keep your mouth shut. Don't even say, "I'll just have a small piece"; that will only draw attention to you. Remember, if you don't make a big deal out of it, the people around you are less likely to. Take the food—small portions if you can manage it—and try to leave some on your plate. Even one bite is a victory, girls. I know I'm advocating wastefulness, God and Grandmom forgive me, but you're got to sacrifice your membership in the clean plate club if you want to be a Former Fat Girl.

Load up on the good stuff.

When there are healthy low-fat and low-cal foods on the menu, load up on these and leave just a little room for the other stuff—green salad, for instance. When I was on my journey, salad became my salvation. I was never a big salad fan before, but I learned that salad was something I could eat in mass quantities without racking up a load of calories. Instead of stuffing my face with pasta or bread or cake, I stuffed my face with salad. While there's no comparison flavorwise, it helped satisfy my drive to eat large amounts of food. Even now when there is salad on the menu at family gatherings (and there usually is because I bring it), I fill at least half my plate with leafy greens so there's only a smidgen of room for the gooey chicken casserole and the cream cheese Jell-O mold. Steamed veggies do the same thing, but I know very few people who serve them without some kind of sauce or at least a good dose of butter (they're just too boring otherwise). Then there are lean meats: They won't fulfill your need for mass quantities, but the protein in them will help satisfy your appetite. Lean cuts of beef, poultry without the skin, fish or shellfish—all are good choices. But watch the preparation method. You're safest with grilled, baked, roasted, or broiled. And exercise caution with fish; many cooks oversauce it so it may be richer than you think.

Lie.

Sometimes the best way to get out of a sticky situation is to fib a little. For instance, say you accepted that piece of cheesecake and managed to take only two bites, as you promised yourself. What do you say when Mom asks why you didn't wolf it down as you normally would? What would it hurt to say you're feeling a little sick to your stomach or feverish or crampy? I don't claim to understand the ways of God, but I don't think he'll damn you for telling such a minor untruth in the spirit of safeguarding yourself from a family firestorm. I've also found that lying can help make restaurant workers take you seriously. Too many times I've ordered a dish without cheese, and it's delivered covered with the stuff. But if I say "I'm allergic to cheese," they get it right four times out of five (which makes me glad I'm not really allergic). If you're concerned about the damage this strategy might do to your soul, I understand (I'm Catholic, after all). Focus your energy on the other tips I've laid out here and whip this one out only as a last resort.

All these tips are working together to give you time to

make your new life a habit. Secret #2 is all about helping you seal yourself off from the influences that might have dragged you down in your weight loss attempts of the past. It protects you from the external distractions—the critical comments, the probing questions, and the spoken and unspoken doubts—so that you can focus on the task at hand: getting healthy, getting fit, and getting stronger and more confident. But what about your inner critic, the voice inside whose favorite words are "you can't" and "never"? The next chapter will reveal the secret to dealing with the saboteur inside.

Chapter Three

Secret #3: Adopt INO: It's Not an Option

I had a mantra before I really even knew what one was. Here's how it all started: I was a pretty good student in high school, getting mostly A's and B's (except for that completely unfair D in trig that I'm still bitter about). I wasn't quite as smart as "The Brains," as we called the kids at the top of the class, but close enough that I counted some of them as friends.

What kept me from superstudent status, I think, was less about pure ability and more about my study habits. Oh, I did my work (a good girl wouldn't slack on homework), but I wasn't the kind of kid who toiled away at the kitchen table late at night agonizing over a paper on some obscure historical event or drilling myself on the anatomy of a fetal pig. No, by 10:00 P.M. I was snoozing.

I just didn't have the drive to excel. Maybe, I think now, it was because of my desire to stay invisible. I couldn't be the kid who won first prize at the science fair or who was chosen to read her A+ essay aloud to the class or who was singled out in any way. I held myself back, afraid of that blinding spotlight that would show every little failure and flaw.

In college, though, I learned to appreciate the value of the all-night study session. It was partly an image thing. I was the only one in my senior class headed to the 2,500-student campus in Austin where I'd chosen to spend my undergraduate years. I saw college as a chance to start over, to shed some of the nerdy image I'd been saddled with since grade school. After all, no one knew me. Oh, anyone could tell by looking at me that I was a Fat Girl, but other than that, there was no preconceived idea of where I belonged in the social structure of the place. At my school there wasn't even all that much of the typical college caste system where the lowly freshmen are not to fraternize with upperclassmen. Plus, no one knew my history. They didn't know, for instance, that the guy who took me to the senior prom got my name off a list of girls who were still dateless three weeks before the dance. (Anyone who was anyone, of course, had a boyfriend or was paired up months in advance.) They didn't hear about the time I started my period in the most obvious way, all over a pair of pale green elastic-waist pants, and walked around the school, oblivious. They might have noticed that I was a Fat Girl—had to, actually—but they didn't seem to quite get what that meant. And that was just fine with me.

It's not like I all of a sudden did a 180 and became some uninhibited, outspoken, take-charge kind of girl with a social calendar as packed as Paris Hilton's. But I did feel more comfortable reaching out to the girls in my dorm and was more receptive to their efforts to reach out to me. It didn't hurt that most of them were in the same situation as I was. They were from all over—New York, Virginia, Florida, and other towns in Texas—and didn't know anyone, either. We all needed one another, so there was less risk of rejection than I'd experienced trying to navigate my clique-heavy high school.

Even so, the last thing I wanted to be pegged was as a nerd, and only a nerd would be organized and conscientious enough to be finished studying in time to get eight hours of sleep the night before a test. No, the cool kids had to cram, and I wanted to be one of the cool kids.

There was a more practical reason, too: The work was harder. I was taking psychology and philosophy, studying Nietzsche and Kierkegaard, and learning about Jung and Freud. Not exactly what you'd call light reading. At my little liberal arts college in the fall of 1978, there was kind of an anything-goes approach to education. There were very few course requirements. I started out thinking that I would major in economics. I had no idea what people who majored in economics did with their lives or even what economics itself actually entailed. I thought it had something to do with government and politics, and I was interested in those things. Econ 101, though, was so excruciatingly boring that I barely made it through the semester, let alone an entire four years. And did I really want to be chairman of the Fed? I don't think so.

Then I thought I'd go pre-law, which is how I found myself reading German philosophers. The actual name of my major is General Studies, which is as close to *whatever* as you can get. I took a lot of the English and philosophy classes that were recommended for pre-law types, but I was able to dabble in a little bit of everything: art history, pottery, psych, computer science, religion, biology, and photography—oh, and PE. I took a tennis class once from the ancient old man who was still coaching well into his eighties. And I vividly remember volleyball class because one day during drills I got slammed in the face with a spike so hard that I thought I had whiplash. I even learned to play racquetball during my college years (it was kind of a craze back then). So I wasn't a complete lump. I tried to get moving, to eat light and eat right, and to get that needle on the scale to move in the desired direction or at least to hold steady. But it wasn't meant to be: I reached my heaviest weight ever just after the end of my senior year.

The obvious reason for my losing battle (how's that for a pun?) was that I had no off switch for my appetite. And there was something else: I'd found myself some partners in crime. Some of my best friends as a freshman—lucky me—were girls who shared my fervor for food, my zeal for meals. What had been my secret shame back home didn't have to be kept secret anymore. As horrible as that shame was, I think it helped rein me in somewhat: sneaking bites under the watchful eyes of my family instead of snuggling up with a whole layer cake out in the open for anyone to see. In the comfort of the dorm, I was free, I was out. My appetite was unleashed.

In fact, probably the most compelling reason for pulling all-nighters with the girls in the dorm was the food. During our many breaks over the course of the evening, we'd raid the lobby vending machine, making a game of trying to steal snacks with a clothes hanger. (Our appetites usually trumped our patience and our skill, and we'd end up pulling out the roll of quarters anyway.) We'd get someone with a car to take us on a Taco Bell run, and I'd order not one but two items: a Bell Beefer with Cheese (a spicy ground beef concoction on a bun, sort of like a sloppy joe) and a Bean Burrito with Cheese. (Do you notice a theme? I was all about the cheese.) When we wanted something sweet, we'd stop by Dunkin' Donuts for an apple fritter the size of a dinner plate. Sometimes we went to the grocery store on the corner for a bag of Nacho Doritos and a six-pack of diet Dr. Pepper (at least it was diet). I couldn't imagine missing out on all the food, er, fun.

But I had a little problem: I wasn't able to keep my eyes open long enough to make it through Johnny Carson's monologue, let alone a 1:00 A.M. food run. I did the usual things to fight off sleep—learned to like coffee, tried No-Doz (and freaked out so badly I never did it again), and even smoked cigarettes, thinking that keeping my hands occupied would help. (It didn't, and I hated the smell.)

Coffee and Cokes helped, but not enough. There had to be something else I could do. So, I kind of started talking to myself. Not in the psychotic-guy-on-the-subway kind of way. I made up something like a mantra that I'd repeat in my head over and over: "Whatever it takes. Whatever it takes. Whatever it takes."

It wasn't just about staying awake to finish my philosophy homework or to have a midnight rendezvous with Ronald McDonald. It was about shutting out the fear that made me give up on myself and go to bed; the fear of excelling, of standing out, of revealing myself, of risking the scrutiny of others. I knew that those few more hours at the books or at the typewriter (this was before PCs) could make a difference in the quality of my work, and I was calling on my inner life coach to get me there. It was as if I had a little Dr. Phil sitting on my shoulder, whispering in my ear: "Whatever it takes."

As silly as that might sound, I was on to something. I started switching on the "Whatever it takes" tape in my head anytime a seemingly impossible deadline loomed: during late nights in the campus newspaper offices laying out the week's edition with only a skeleton staff to help; writing my fifty-plus-page senior thesis. I found myself not giving up so easily and starting to excel both in the classroom and outside of it. This mantra, coupled with the more nurturing and accepting environment of my college campus, gave me the push I needed to put myself out there little by little once again. I started getting involved in campus activities—on the yearbook staff, in student government, and on the newspaper. This was a very small place, remember. There was a core group of about twenty students who did just about everything on campus, and I became one of them. But you didn't really have to do much more than show up to earn it. Larger schools, such as the University of Texas where I got my master's, were far more competitive. Student government campaigns are more sophisticated there than the legislative races in Alabama where I now live (which might not be saying all that much). In that cutthroat setting I would have needed more than a mantra to get me to step into the fray.

"Whatever it takes" helped me inch out of my shell academically but only to a point socially. Sure, I became one of the "doers" on campus and accumulated a good group of girlfriends, but what about the boys? I haven't mentioned any (except the poor guy who took me to the prom) because there *weren't* any. Seriously. My senior year of college I could still count on one hand the number of guys I'd even kissed, with the exception of relatives. I didn't even have a first date until my junior year in high school. George was one of two guys in the group I hung around with, and I think he "dated" every one of us at least once. I'm not sure why he all of a sudden latched on to me; I think it was just my turn. Anyway, we went to dinner and faked our way into a dance club where we swayed to Lionel Ritchie's "Once, Twice, Three Times a Lady" (I'm cringing with embarrassment even now). And, yes, we made out in his car—kissing only. I was sixteen and had never made out before. (How proud my mom must be reading this!)

Oh, I had crushes, but not on George. No, I thought there must be something wrong with him if he actually liked me, or there was some other motive at work (that it was just my turn, as I mentioned before). Any guy I even suspected of being attracted to me, and there weren't many, had to be flawed.

You know how that is: Only someone warped could think that you, Fat Girl you, would be any more than a pal. Even that is a stretch. Because how could anyone else bear to look at you long enough to have a conversation when you can't even stand to look at yourself in the mirror? And that's fully clothed. Naked? Not even a possibility.

No, my secret crush in high school was John, the other guy in my circle of friends. He was dating one of the girls in our group, and I think on some level that's why I picked him. He was safe. After all, I would never betray a friend by making a move on her guy. A great excuse for not risking my heart, isn't it? How noble of me.

Even when he and my friend Katie were on the outs, which they were regularly, there was never any real danger that he would get too close. I made sure of that. In my Fat Girl way I had made him more of a buddy than a boyfriend. With him I became like one of the guys, cracking jokes, swearing like a sailor, showing off my smarts—almost posturing like guys do. I didn't know any other way to be with guys. After all, that's how I related to my brothers and (with the exception of the swearing part) my dad.

I'm now convinced that my Fat Girl programming kept my heart sealed off from any kind of intimate relationship with a man. I just couldn't conceive of the idea that any guy in his right mind could be attracted to me. The funny thing was, during the height of my crush on John, my weight was actually at a low point. I was playing tennis semiregularly (partly because John did), and I had taken to running at night with my little dog, Daisy. But I couldn't seem to shake that Fat Girl mentality.

For years I managed to effectively neuter the rare guy who showed interest in me as anything more than a buddy; I cluelessly sucked all the sexuality and sensuality out of the relationship. I just didn't know any other way. I was oblivious to even the most overt expressions of interest from a guy. For instance, when I was a senior in college—and my weight had shot back up almost as high as it would ever go—there was a freshman who kind of followed me around like a puppy dog. I didn't think twice about the fact that he always seemed to be hanging out in the student newspaper offices where, as editor, I also spent a lot of time. One day one of the other editors referred to "the crush" Kevin had on me as if it were common knowledge. I scoffed and quickly found a reason to leave the room. I remember actually thinking, "How could he like me? I'm *fat!*" With that attitude, no wonder I was always the friend, never the girlfriend.

It would be years before I experienced any kind of breakthrough in the romance department. (Don't worry, you'll get the details later.) But there was no denying that "Whatever it takes" was a pretty powerful tool. After all, it had helped me begin to push beyond the Fat Girl limits I'd set for myself, the limits that kept me stuck in mediocrity.

Early in my journey toward becoming a Former Fat Girl I began wondering whether some kind of mantra could get me through the sessions at the track when I'd rather be anywhere else, or the times when the dessert cart was staring me in the face, just begging for me to take the bait.

·It was during one of my seemingly interminable runs around the dusty track I had begun to frequent that it came to me. I was at around lap eight when the whiner in my head started doing her thing. "Can't we quit now? Pleeeeeze?" she asked. "After all, we've made it through two whole miles. That's like fourteen in the Fat Girl time/space continuum, right?"

For a second there I almost gave in. Two miles was pretty good, damn good. But no—I'd planned to do three miles, and that meant I had four more laps to go. I was playing a game of mental tug-of-war with that stubborn inner whiner when it popped out: "It's not an option," I said to myself.

And there it was.

Those four little words ended the internal argument right there. The effect was like a steel door slamming shut in an empty warehouse. It had such a finality to it, you could almost hear the echo. "It's not an option." With that phrase I'd shut off a whole world of possibility, a world where giving up was not just acceptable but the norm.

I got through the full three miles that night, blurting out "It's not an option" every time the whiner started making noises about quitting. Soon after, I started using "It's not an option" (INO, for short) to get my butt to the track every day. That's right—every single day. Skip a session? INO. I didn't trust myself early on to take even a day of rest; it would be too easy, I feared, to get sucked back into my old sedentary routine. I wanted exercise to become routine. I wanted to need it as much as I needed to brush my teeth in the morning or put in my contacts. I wanted to feel odd, off-kilter, almost unable to function without it.

Obsessive? Maybe. Okay, definitely. I didn't know it at the time, but I was merely swapping one obsession for another. As a Fat Girl, I'd been obsessed with food my whole life. My mind was filled with thoughts of food, and I needed something else to occupy my brain cells. Exercise—running, to be specific—was it.

Because of INO, I ran in the rain, I suffered on the treadmill, and I wrenched myself out of bed in the early morning if I knew I wouldn't be able to run after work. INO helped me kick food off the top spot on my list of priorities. There was a new object of my obsession. And it felt *good*.

INO was just as effective when I finally did take on my diet about three years into my Former Fat Girl quest. By that time my exercise obsession had already carved me down from a size 16 or so to a size 8. Then, for reasons I'll explain later, I decided to go on Weight Watchers.

The Weight Watchers of the mid-80s was a bit different than it is now. You were allowed a certain number of servings from the different food groups: breads/grains, dairy, meat/protein, fruits/vegetables. Every time you ate a serving from a group, you'd mark it down. Once you exhausted, say, your six-serving bread/grain quota (which I could do before noon), that was it. No more bread that day. You were forced to tap the other food groups for the rest of the day's meals. In that way the program actually compelled you to eat a balanced diet. Today's version is somewhat looser. You're given a set number of "points" each day and a guide to how many points a serving of each food will set you back. If you choose to, you could spend your whole day's worth of points on chocolate (hmmm, I see a new ad campaign in Weight Watchers' future). Then again, that would tap you out pretty fast, and you'd be left sampling from the zero-point menu: ice cubes, water, diet drinks, and Splenda. Yum.

People often say Weight Watchers—both the ancient version I was on and the modern one—teaches you portion control. The portion part I buy. WW had me weighing my breakfast cereal with a tiny little kitchen scale, parceling out sliced strawberries in a cup measure, and making note of the number of ounces in a yogurt container. Don't get me wrong: That was a big lesson for a girl who was used to eating a half pound of pasta at one sitting (and toying with the idea of going back for seconds).

The "control" part, though, has to come from you. After all, you're the one who has to put on the brakes when the bread basket's sitting there, overflowing, within reach. You're the one who has to resist rummaging through the pantry for a midnight snack when you've already maxed out your points for the day. You're the one who has to fight back all those inbred urges that make you want to eat when you aren't even hungry anymore.

For me that's where INO came in. Whenever I was tempted to stray beyond the limits of the WW diet, I whipped out INO. Again, I was superstrict about it. A slice of pizza? INO. Even though a mere slice wouldn't have broken the WW bank, I couldn't rely on myself to stop at one. An after-work beer? INO. I knew myself well enough to know that I wouldn't be able to resist a refill and the nachos, nuts, or whatever other bar food found its way to the table. A slice of cake, even just a bite? INO. Not for this sugar addict.

"It's not an option" helped me take the boundaries set for me by the Weight Watchers diet and the boundaries I'd set for myself exercisewise and make them mean something. Until I discovered INO, it was anything goes; the rule was there were no rules. I could eat anything, do nothing, or eat nothing, do everything, whatever. If I was to become a Former Fat Girl, that had to stop. For me INO was like putting blinders on a race horse: It helped block out all the distractions and kept my eyes trained on what lay ahead.

If you have any doubts about the power of INO to change your life, think about this: Right now other "mere words" have just as much power over you. Words like "I am weak" and "I am not worthy." Words like "I can't" and "I will always be a Fat Girl." These words are defining you; they are shaping the way you live now. Secret #3: Adopt INO (It's Not an Option) can help you fix all that.

Chant Like a Former Fat Girl

INO will help you do the thing that beyond anything else you must do to become a Former Fat Girl—and it could be the most difficult—and that is to say no. You're working against years of Fat Girl programming that has you thinking you're incapable of refusing that second piece of cake even though you're not hungry for it. Your appetite has trumped your willpower for so long that you don't believe you can turn the tables.

Even more than that, INO gives you a way of saying no to the people and responsibilities you automatically put ahead of yourself and your own needs. It gives you permission to put yourself first, an essential step toward Former Fat Girlhood. Using it as a tool, you can rearrange your priorities and elevate yourself to the proper position on your to-do list: the top.

INO was invaluable in helping me overcome my need to please and my talent for rationalizing that putting other people first—just about at all cost—was somehow the noble thing to do. It helped me say no when the demands of family and friends threatened to disrupt my running routine; it helped me say no to seconds of Mom's cheesy, oozing lasagna even though I knew such a rebuff might hurt her feelings. It helped give me the courage to break out of the Fat Girl mold that other people expected me to conform to, and start living my own way.

When I think about it now, I wasn't as much putting others *before* me as I was putting myself *last*. That might seem like a game of semantics, but it's not. My lack of self-confidence and self-respect made me feel like I didn't deserve to be first. As I worked the Former Fat Girl program, as I began to re-shape my self-image, I began to see that for me to get what I wanted in life, to get anywhere other than where I was, I had to put my needs first. And INO helped make it happen.

To use INO you have to define the rules of your new life. How often do you want to exercise? What are you trying to do with your diet? Once you have some kind of plan, INO can help you follow it. I know what you're thinking: "Ugh. Another diet? Another exercise program? Just what I need." I promise—that's not what I'm talking about here. Where you get your "rules" is up to you. You might be the kind of person who grooves on a cookie-cutter program that someone else sets out for you. Chances are, though, that you've cycled through your share of those, and if they lived up to their hype, you wouldn't be reading this book. But I don't believe in re-grets. With every crazy diet you've been on, you've learned something about yourself, something that will help you figure out what *will* work for you. The challenge is tapping that knowledge. That's what I'm here to help you with.

The idea of living (and eating) by some set of rules yet again is hard to even think about, I know. When your life is so full of stress (as most of ours are), you savor the freedom to eat what you want and do what you want with the little downtime you have. Indulging your appetite for food, for mindless TV watching, for lounging and leisure might be the only way you nurture yourself. And the last thing I want to do is deny you that. But you know on some level that the overeating and inactivity are hurting you more than helping you. Any sense of comfort that these things give you is false. Rather than nurturing your spirit, they're sapping your strength. They are what's standing between you and the life you want.

Once you know your new limits, you have to find a way to nurture yourself within them. It's a delicate balance: You must be firm enough with yourself to put into place the changes that will make you a Former Fat Girl, but not so by-the-book that you drive yourself back to the same old patterns that held you down before. How do you strike that balance? These Former Fat Girl Fixes will help.

The Obstacle: Knowing What Your Rules Should Be

A new weight loss theory is born every minute. Okay, so I made that up, but it's not too far from the truth. There's a lot of crazy, confusing advice about the right way to eat and exercise. When you set out to create the rules for your new life, what advice do you follow?

Former Fat Girl Fixes

List the rules you eat by now.

Before you go all knee-jerk on me and say, "I thought the problem is that I don't *have* any," think for a minute. There are patterns to the way you eat and the way you behave that are probably not working for you. I, for instance, always had a snack at around 3:00 P.M., no question. It didn't matter if I had a three-course lunch; the snack was just something I did (and it wasn't some virtuous piece of fruit—more like a Snickers or a bag of Doritos). Here's another one: When I had spaghetti, my bowl had to be filled to where the blue pattern started on the rim. Anything less just wasn't enough. I never asked myself if I really wanted that snack or that much pasta. Those were my unconscious rules, and there were others: It was okay to have seconds on anything as long as my mom and dad would let me. I could order dessert if other people were ordering dessert. I could even order two if other people were ordering two. Sandwiches always had cheese on them. Pizza always had pepperoni. There was no such thing as just one cookie, just one potato chip, or just one bite. Plates were always cleaned unless they contained anything green, peas and lima beans in particular. Get the picture?

The first step in making INO work for you is to get in touch with the rules you're living by now. Here's how: Pull out a sheet of paper and write fifteen statements that begin with the words "I always" or "I never." Include anything related to your relationship with food. Why fifteen? Because I want you to stretch, to make yourself really examine what you might be doing that threatens to sabotage you on your way to becoming a Former Fat Girl. If you hit fifteen easily, go for twenty. If twenty is easy, go for twenty-five. You may need to give yourself a couple of days or even a week to get a good list together. Different rules can emerge in different situations (at work, at leisure, in social activities, and so on). Push yourself. Get it all out there—because you can't create new rules unless you know what the old ones are.

Tap your inner diet database.

If you're a veteran of as many weight loss plans as I am, you have a wealth of information in your head that could help you on your journey to Former Fat Girlhood. For instance, if you were ever on Atkins or Sugar Busters, you know how you pined for a thick piece of sourdough bread or a nice potato (white, please). If you ever took the super-low-fat route, you know how sick you got of that rubbery stuff they call fat-free cheese. If South Beach was your plan of choice, you know how poorly your number-phobic brain handled the whole GI index thing. You might already know from past experience what you hate about treadmill walking or that you can't stand exercising when it gets below 57.4 degrees outside. I'll bet you learned some positive things, too, like the fact that music can make just about any type of exercise more tolerable but only if it's R&B (no disco or classic rock for you). Or maybe you didn't mind having just that Slim-Fast shake for breakfast, but what tripped you up was that you needed a lunch you could actually chew. Or maybe going without dessert during the week wasn't so bad but you really missed it on the weekends when you were ready to live a little.

To get to all that data, here's another little exercise. At the top of a blank sheet of paper, write down the name of a weight loss regimen you tried in the past—a diet, an exercise routine, what have you. Then list at least three things about the program that worked for you and at least three things that didn't. Do that for each of the different approaches you've tried (three to five ought to be enough). Include programs of your own creation as well—say, for instance, the month you had only soup for breakfast, lunch, and dinner. Again, stretch yourself. The "didn't work" column will probably be easy for you to fill up; feel free to list more than three. The stuff that worked will likely be a struggle to come up with; force yourself to list at least three, and if that's easy, come up with a few more. This is the second step in creating a set of rules that will get you to your Former Fat Girl goal, rules that you can stick with (helped by INO) for the long haul.

Turn the information into action.

Take your fifteen rules (or whatever number you end up with) and choose two diet-related rules to tackle. Then shuffle through your diet database to see if you jotted down any past experiences that relate to how you should rewrite those rules. It is easier than it sounds. For instance, from my database, I know that the times when I tried to skip my 3:00 P.M. snack altogether—especially during the workweek—were disastrous. I found that not only did I need the snack to help hold me until dinner (otherwise, I'd go right for the cookie jar when I set foot in the house), but my brain needed the break. So instead of just cutting myself off completely, I rewrote the rule this way: "I always have a piece of fruit or a small bag of pretzels at 3:00 P.M. during the workweek." And then when I was tempted to grab a candy bar or a piece of leftover birthday cake instead, I activated my INO mechanism.

If you think this is no big deal, let's look at the impact. First, the physical: A vending machine bag of pretzels is about 120 calories; a pack of Oreos from that same machine is 200.

Eating the pretzels instead of the Oreos five days a week saves me 400 calories; skipping the snack altogether on the weekends (because I don't really miss it then) saves me another 400. That's 800 calories a week saved; over a year, that's a grand total of 41,600 calories. It takes 3,500 calories to equal 1 pound of body fat, so with this little no-brainer strategy, you'd lose almost 12 pounds over the course of a year! (Okay, so it's 11.8857 pounds for you sticklers, but that's still pretty good.)

The emotional benefit is immeasurable but just as powerful. Every time you choose those pretzels over those Oreos or follow your new rule instead of the old one, you'll see the needle on that self-esteem scale move in the right direction. Choosing that salty snack is like saying yes to the Former Fat Girl way of life and leaving the Fat Girl you used to be sitting in the queue, like the Oreos, growing stale and moldy by the minute.

Give yourself six weeks to get those two new rules down, and then add another. Resist the urge to move too fast. Allow yourself time to get comfortable living by these new rules and use INO to keep you honest.

What about exercise?

You're not off the hook. In addition to the two diet-related rules you're going to tackle, you need to come up with one exercise-related rule. The process is a little different, though. Chances are you don't have any rules about exercise now, so you have to start from scratch. A good beginner's goal is to shoot for thirty minutes three days a week. That works out to about every other day, which is regular enough for you to get used to but not so demanding that it's extraordinarily hard to accommodate. (If you have preexisting health problems, are severely overweight, or simply would feel more secure with a professional's blessing, talk to your doctor before you commit to a goal.)

Wait a minute. Didn't I say I had to run every day to make sure I didn't slip back into the life of a sloth? Yes, but when I first started exercising, I was doing Jazzercise only three days a week. I didn't jump right in and commit to a seven-day running regimen. I took my baby steps, too. The point is to start establishing exercise as a habit, to commit to some regular schedule and, with the help of INO, make it permanent. Also, the information you have in your diet database—what you've learned about yourself from trying fitness-related programs in the past—will help you screen out activities and situations that might get in the way of achieving your three-days-a-week goal. Use that and the Former Fat Girl Fixes from chapter 1 to help you write an exercise rule you can keep.

Don't be afraid to revise.

Now, I don't have to tell you that living by these new rules won't be easy. You can well imagine my anguish, I'm sure, at leaving those delicious Oreos to rot in the vending machine. No matter how tough it is, stick it out for those six weeks. At the end of that time, reassess. If feelings of denial, temptation, despair, or whatever are trumping the self-esteem booster shot you should be getting from sticking with your program for this long, you may need to take another look at the rules you've been working with. Take my pretzel-versus-Oreo scenario, for example: Maybe I find that I do need the Saturday and Sunday 3:00 P.M. snack after all. Or, maybe I miss those Oreos so much that I allow myself to have them on Monday afternoons following the weekly staff meeting that always seems to bring me down. Rigidity is what dooms most cookie-cutter diets in the first place, but too much flexibility won't get you where you want to be, either.

The Obstacle: Feelings of Deprivation That Threaten to Throw You Off Track

INO can keep you going through a tough workout or help you pass up a gratuitous piece of chocolate, but let's get real: It doesn't sound like very much fun. I've got the fixes for that.

Former Fat Girl Fixes

Know when to use INO and when not to.

INO is not meant to be an iron rule. Use it too often, and you could start having flashbacks to old weight loss attempts when you walked around feeling deprived of food, of fun, of all the good things in life. As valuable as INO can be to future Former Fat Girls like you, to get the most out of it you have to know when to use it. For instance, I don't believe that it applies to eating a piece of your son's, your husband's or your own birthday cake. But the cheap Wal-Mart cupcakes at the office party for the payroll secretary you don't even like? INO. Try sorting through scenarios like that to determine INO-appropriate situations. And by all means, if you start having those flashbacks, take a look at how you're using INO and pull back if you need to.

Build in some free-food time.

There is a way to preserve some of the freedom you loved when you allowed yourself to eat whatever you wanted whenever you wanted it. All you need to do is set aside some situations where you can take that free and easy approach. I've used several techniques for this. A particular favorite, one that I still use today, is to limit my breakfast and lunch options to one or

Three Questions to Ask Yourself Before Using INO

You already know that INO is a powerful weapon. It's like the psychological equivalent of an Uzi: It'll riddle those temptations and those excuses with holes, but you have to use it right or you'll shoot yourself in the foot. (Whew! Some metaphor, eh?) Quiz yourself before you fire away.

1. **Is the rule I'm trying to follow realistic?** If you try to use INO to help you keep some kind of impossible commitment, you're doomed to fail. Here's one: "I will never eat dessert again." Now, what normal person could keep that promise? You want rules that will challenge you but that you don't have to be incarcerated or dead to keep.

2. **Am I sick?** Okay, this is the whole "listen to your body" speech. Sometimes it's simply better for you to skip a workout, like when you have the flu or you are completely exhausted or have a pain in your knee that won't go away. But be tough on yourself. You know how your body likes to take the easy way out.

3. **Am I obsessed in a bad way?** As I've already explained, I was somewhat obsessive about my running routine early

on. I think that's actually necessary if you're trying to re-program yourself—but it shouldn't be done to the point where you're risking your job, hurting friends, family, or yourself, or shirking other responsibilities. These are red flags that you're taking your program too far. If that's the case, please see your doctor and get help before you find yourself in real trouble.

two dishes so that I can have more freedom at dinner. For instance, breakfast is oatmeal five days a week and a bagel with light cream cheese (an indulgence) on the weekends; lunch is a half sandwich or bowl of soup. Dinner could be more substantial: chicken tacos with guacamole, pad Thai, or salmon, baked potato, and salad. That technique keeps my calories in check and feeds my need for an interesting evening meal that my whole family can get into. It also gives my diet some structure, but not so much that I'm constantly battling the temptation to break the rules. Plus, the monotony of breakfast and lunch makes dinner seem even more special.

You could also make your weekdays more structured and allow yourself more freedom on the weekends. I used that approach when I was single. It was more important for me to go out and indulge on the weekends; I didn't mind eating lighter during the workweek. One more idea: At one point in my life, in my late twenties, I had really strong cravings for sweets and other carbs during my period. If I had a taste for something, I was like a madwoman; it was worse than any craving I had years later when I was pregnant with my son. I decided I would allow myself one day where I could eat anything I wanted in any quantity. I had figured out that my cravings were the most intense the day after I started my period, so that became what I called my free day. I remember one time when I was dying for a peanut butter–chocolate chip cookie. It was nearing the official end of my free day—midnight—and I found an open store that happened to have such a confection. I ate it, but it wasn't quite right; it wasn't *the* peanut butter–chocolate chip cookie that my taste buds were yearning for. I think I went to every convenience store in Austin that night searching, unembarrassed, for that perfect cookie, sampling many along the way. But at the stroke of midnight it was over, and I was back to INO. Even though I was drawn to that perfect cookie like a magnet to metal, INO helped me defy the laws of physics and keep my Former Fat Girl commitment.

Preserve your perspective.

How *not* to use INO: to make yourself feel bad for not living up to some impossible standard you set for yourself. Think about INO as the encouraging words of a coach, not the judgmental command of a drill sergeant. It is meant to lift you up, not tear you down. Respect yourself for every little bit of progress you make. You deserve it.

The Obstacle: Lack of Time, the Mother of All Excuses

Time is second only to "I don't like it" on the list of reasons that women don't exercise. How can you even think INO could help you make exercise a priority when you can't find the time to send your own mother a birthday card or make the bed in the morning? Wait—check out my fixes.

Former Fat Girl Fixes

Move whenever you can.

You don't have hours to spend in the gym. Who does? How can you be expected to listen to the INO in your head and squeeze in a workout on the days when every minute is committed to someone or something else? As insurance when it's just not possible to get to the gym or the trail, seize any opportunity to move during the day. Don't scoff. I know you've

No Time? No Excuse: How to Find the Time You Need to Take Care of You

You may be thinking, "Use INO to help keep me exercising? Maybe if I had, like, a whole different life. There already aren't enough hours in the day!" Hey, I know what you mean. I used to think that, too. Here's how to shortcut that excuse:

1. Repeat after me: How I spend my time is *my choice*. Post it on your computer monitor, keep it in your planner, write it on the back of your hand (remember when you used to do that?)—anything to remind you.

2. Map out how you spent your time over the past week. Be as detailed as you possibly can about your hours outside of work. For instance, instead of saying "housework," say "dusted the living room, folded clothes." Instead of saying "watched TV," list the shows. Do that for each day of the week.

3. Highlight *productive time* in yellow. By *productive time* I mean housework, helping kids with homework, taking care of other family members, shopping for necessities (versus leisure shopping), and so on—anything you consider part of your job as an adult.

4. Highlight *enrichment time* in blue. By that I mean time you spend reading, practicing a hobby, learning something new,

exercising, and so forth—anything you find refreshing or fulfilling.

5. Highlight *entertainment time* in pink. Going to movies, watching TV, listening to music, and eating out—all are considered entertainment time. Include only activities you truly enjoyed. If you were sitting, bored, in front of the TV, that doesn't count.

6. Look for any blocks of time that you didn't highlight. That's the no-brainer way to find time in your schedule. If you're not doing something productive, enriching, or entertaining, what else is there? Could you be using this time to, say, exercise?

7. Look at the proportion of your time that's highlighted yellow. There's a good chance you don't have any nonhighlighted areas and that you have a whole lot of yellow on your map. Fat Girls have a way of taking on an inordinate amount of responsibility, probably because it helps make us feel loved when we believe we are so unlovable. To reach your goal of becoming a Former Fat Girl, you have to shift some of those tasks to other people. You have to ask for help and leave some things undone. Start by asking for help with one task—maybe grocery shopping (because the food store is not a great place for you) or laundry. Little by little you'll be more comfortable with sharing the responsibilities you've shouldered for so long. Oh, and you'll start to find time for some of those things you've been wanting to do for yourself—like that thirty-minute treadmill walk.

heard this before, but I wouldn't repeat it if I didn't know that it will make a difference. If you take the stairs instead of the elevator, walk instead of drive (when possible), and even stand instead of sit, you'll burn more calories in the course of the day. That's not a great substitute for a sweaty session on the elliptical trainer, but it gives you some cushion when other commitments outrank you and your workouts on your list of priorities. So INO to use the elevator unless you're wearing three-inch heels or your doctor says you can't for some reason. And if you're using the heels as an excuse, ditch them for flats. They're easier to walk in, better for your feet, and back in style, too.

Split it up.

Can't find 30 minutes for a good treadmill walk? What about 15? Or 10? Research says that short bursts of exercise are just as effective as one long session. If you can't imagine getting up early enough to do a 30-minute walk in the morning, try 15 minutes then and 15 minutes when you get home from work. Or if you can walk at lunch, do three 10-minute segments. This strategy works best for walkers and people with home exercise equipment such as treadmills, bikes, and elliptical trainers.

Don't do nothing.

My grammatically correct grandmother is turning in her grave, but this situation calls for a double negative: Doing *something* physical is always better than doing nothing at all. Absolutely can't squeeze in thirty minutes on the treadmill? Fifteen minutes isn't so bad. Miss the start of your cycling class at the gym? Jump on a bike in the cardio room for twenty minutes. Lunchtime walk rained out? Climb the stairs in your office building for twenty minutes instead. Too many times, people let a glitch in their system throw them completely off track. Don't give in to that temptation.

Quit being a martyr.

My psychologist friend Alice Domar, Ph.D., has a much nicer term for it: self-sacrificer. The theory is that you really do have the time you need to do right by your body and your mind. But I say that because of your Fat Girl programming, you don't feel worthy of the top spot on your to-do list. Your name is inked in, typeset, right there at the bottom. So, naturally, everyone else and everything else defaults to a position ahead of you.

The first step in elevating yourself in your own eyes is to recognize that for the most part your so-called lack of time is the result of your own choices. You are choosing to put other people's needs above your own. Sure, you have housework to do and kids to care for—hey, we all do. But has it ever occurred to you that you could ask others to take on some of those tasks? Probably not, because that's part of the Fat Girl programming. Everyone else's "stuff" is more important than yours. To be a Former Fat Girl you have to stop thinking that way, stop self-sacrificing. To help give you a visual picture of how you're spending your time—and where you might find more time for you—see the sidebar on page 100.

I can't tell you how much of a difference INO has made in my life, in the way I deal with food, in my commitment to exercise, and even in the decisions I make every day. Whereas I used to swallow my discontent, my creative ideas, my clever quips, now It's Not an Option *not* to. That mantra is one of the central themes of my life even now, after all these years. It keeps me going, day after day, helping me resist my self-sacrificing tendencies, my self-doubts, the temptation to sleep in, to pig out, to give up on myself.

While Secret #3 was about how to get to where you want to be physically and emotionally, Secret #4 will help you figure out how to know when you've actually arrived. It's designed to help you confront the assumptions and fears that have kept you stuck in your comfort zone and create a clear picture of what it means to be a Former Fat Girl: how you want to look, how you want to feel, how you want to act in the world. A tall order, I know, but it can be done. Read on to find out how.

Chapter Four

Secret #4: "See" Yourself Slim

I had done it. By focusing on fitness and not on dieting, by keeping my nascent Former Fat Girl journey secret from the people around me, and by using the INO mantra to stay focused and put myself first on my to-do list, I had dropped from a size 16-plus to about an 8. And I thought that's where my big-boned body was meant to be.

Not only that, I had started wrenching myself little by little out of the safe, comfortable cocoon of a life I had created. After all, I had always been afraid of moving on, of taking the next step. As a kid I moped around on Sunday afternoons, dreading the beginning of the school week; I literally mourned the end of summer break. When all my friends were dying to get their driver's permit at fifteen, I was happy to wait until seventeen, delaying that rite of passage as long as I could. As an adult, college graduation represented the end of another long, long summer for me. The campus was my home, my haven, and I didn't want to leave.

I had started to flourish there, indulging the overachiever in me like I was never able to do in my politically cutthroat high school. I was like Forrest Gump, popping up in almost every scene—tutoring underclassmen, working on any and every campus committee, cheering in the stands at all the basketball games (that is, if I wasn't taking photos for the newspaper), and planning student retreats. My status as *über*volunteer earned me the school's ultimate prize, Woman of the Year, given to the graduating senior with the longest list of extracurricular activities. No one else came close.

I did all this at the expense of my own schoolwork: Heading into my last week of classes as a senior, I remember having four research papers due, and I had yet to start even one. That was status quo for me throughout college, to spread myself so thin that I was sick with anxiety as finals approached and rushed to catch up—sick in the literal sense with symptoms that always seemed to strike a couple of weeks before finals: stomach cramps that had me running for the john, a heart racing so fast that I thought it would leap out of my chest, and backaches that left me sleepless when I finally did make it to bed after a late-night cramming session.

I was carrying such a heavy load, and I'm not talking about the eighteen class hours I took most semesters. With every activity I got into, I sucked up responsibility like a sponge. If something went wrong—a missed deadline, a low turnout at student elections, a typo in a front-page story—it was my fault, or so I thought, even if the mishap was completely out of my control. I was the one who took up the slack if anyone else didn't come through, which seemed to happen a lot, probably because everyone knew I was there, ready to come to the rescue.

I always managed to get my academic work done, though, and done well enough to make the dean's list most semesters. Looking back, I think I was hooked on the whole drama of it: *Would Lisa manage to pull off leading the end-of-the-semester retreat, close the last issue of the newspaper,* and *take three finals and write four papers in one week? Or will she self destruct under all the pressure? Tune in next week to find out.*

But more than that, I loved being the go-to girl, the one everyone could count on. I wore my busyness like a badge of honor and took pride in my packed schedule. Getting an actual award for it made me wriggle with delight inside, like a dog that just can't wag its tail hard enough. I didn't even mind the glare of the spotlight as I walked across the stage in front of applauding family, friends, and faculty to pick up my walnut plaque with the engraved brass plate. All the praise, the applause, and the gratitude made the work worthwhile and made me feel worthy. To this people-pleaser, it was like winning an Academy Award.

The idea of leaving all this was terrifying—much scarier to me than going from high school to college. In high school I never even had a chance at the kind of go-to-girl status I had attained in college; that was reserved for only the most popular kids in the tightest cliques. Graduation meant I would have to start over somewhere else, tiptoeing around and testing the waters, figuring out whether I could speak my mind without getting shut down, figuring out who was friend and who was foe, figuring out how to please and whom to please. Graduation meant I had to find my place again.

But I couldn't stay. I took too much pride in my smarts to be one of those students who kept delaying graduation, taking one more class, tackling one more major, so I did the next best thing: I signed up to get a master's in journalism at the University of Texas across town. The booming forty-thousand-student campus was like New York City compared to my tiny school, but it was still college, where A's were good and F's were bad, where the professors ruled. Not like the murky corporate world, full of unknown enemies, unclear politics, and often incomprehensible measures of success. Familiar territory, or more familiar than some cubicle in an office building downtown.

And, anyway, I rationalized, how did I even think I could be a journalist with my measly General Studies degree? Never mind that I had been editor of the weekly campus newspaper. Never mind that I probably had as much experience, if not more, than kids whose transcripts were full of classes in reporting and editing. In my mind there was no way I could measure up.

It wasn't until I started my whole Former Fat Girl journey a year into grad school that I began to see that many of the choices I'd made in life were made out of fear. That my fear of rejection had kept me from striking out on my own, away from the arms of academia. That I was so afraid that if I stopped giving, giving, giving—to the point that I didn't even know what I wanted for myself—there would be no more reason for my parents, my professors, or my peers to love me. That fear was what kept me from loving any guy who was free to love me back, as much because he *might* as because he *might not*. That fear was the real reason I couldn't shed the pounds I had been battling for so many years.

I was just as afraid of success as I was of failure. By not trying for the kind of job I dreamed of, I didn't have to face the idea that maybe I wasn't as smart or as creative as I thought. By not trying for the available guy and instead secretly pining for the boyfriend of a best friend, I was insulating myself from rejection. I was also protecting myself from the reality of relationships in all their complicated, messy imperfection. I preferred the perfection of my daydream trysts to the prospect of finding out that he (whoever he might be) wasn't perfect, that *I* wasn't perfect. And by remaining apart, by maintaining my buddy status, I was shielding myself from the real pain of losing someone I had allowed into my world. Losing a buddy is like pulling off a hangnail; losing a lover is like yanking out a molar sans anesthesia.

And if I lost the weight, I'd lose the perfect fallback excuse for the times I did try and failed: *Of course he doesn't want me— I'm fat!*

It was like that excess seventyish pounds was some kind of impenetrable armor. Shedding it would leave me exposed, vulnerable to ridicule, to teasing, and to all the associated pain. I know it doesn't sound rational. I was teased as a Fat Girl, but I was afraid to lose weight because I might be teased for *not* being fat? I think I had become so familiar with my Fat Girl role that I was afraid of *any* change.

Now this was a different ball game. For years I had thought that if I could just find the right diet—the perfect scientific ratio of fat to carbs to protein to whatever—I could get that "perfect" body. I thought that if I wasn't such a weakling, I could resist those Girl Scout Thin Mints calling to me from the pantry.

I wasn't completely wrong about the weakling part. I did have to build my physical and mental strength to break out of that Fat Girl mode, but I figured out that I was fighting the wrong enemy. Instead of focusing on my appetite, I needed to set my sights on that fear—the fear that was keeping the needle on the scale stuck in the "heavy" position, the fear that was ruling my life in all kinds of ways.

I kind of backed into this whole revelation about the fear factor as I made it through each workout and saw the payoffs on the scale. I began to feel a little surge of strength inside and outside after every run around that quarter-mile track and every time I made it through the day without pigging out. I felt brave enough to push a little further during the next workout, more confident that I could resist the temptations of the treats I so loved. I started looking forward to the next thing instead of down at my feet, like you do out of shame, out of shyness, out of insecurity. And I had more energy to actually move toward it.

As I cast off my "fat clothes," there were signs that I was beginning to shed the Fat Girl image I had of myself. For one thing, I started experimenting with my wardrobe, my hair, and my makeup. You know something's going on when a Fat Girl actually looks forward to shopping. Trying on clothes was becoming less of a self-esteem-sucking experience and more like something out of *Goldilocks and the Three Bears*: These pants? Too tight. This pair? Too loose. This one? Just right. Before, there *was* no "just right." I'd had a closet full of supersize clothes, but I didn't feel "just right" in any of them. Now, even though I still experienced my share of dressing room disappointments, I was a little more confident that there was a "just right" somewhere on the rack waiting for me. Shopping for my size 8 body was—dare I say?—*fun*.

This was back in the 80s when Boy George-ish androgyny was in: Everyone was wearing oversized, straight-cut, double-breasted suit jackets with baggy, pleated, menswear-inspired pants. I was particularly fond of the stretchy-stirrup-pants-with-big-sweater look. I took to wearing the occasional tie, like everyone else. I remember a particular wardrobe favorite, a linen-cotton blend suit jacket in a rust color with a khaki pinstripe. The shoulder pads were thicker than a sofa cushion. In it I looked like a gangster at a Gatsby garden party.

Hey, I never said the clothes were tasteful, but I loved them anyway. I hadn't felt this way about anything in my wardrobe since the white vinyl go-go boots I begged my dad to buy me on one of our father-daughter shopping trips when I was a little girl. And the fact that I even *cared*, even *dared* to dip my big toe into the deep blue sea of fashion was pretty amazing. For years my size had kept me from wearing what everyone else was wearing. Now more than ever before I was on trend. I even developed a fetish for chunky earrings, the chunkier and funkier the better. I invested in a palette of eye shadows worthy of a movie-set makeup artist, applying no less than three shades (and sometimes more) in combination. I wore *lipstick*, for God's sake.

Before, my only fashion goal had been to fade into the background; now, I wanted to be *noticed*.

Even so, a struggle was going on beneath the surface of my Debbie Gibson-esque exterior. With every step I took toward the spotlight, I had to fight back the old Fat Girl fears that had kept me in hiding for so long. Every change I made on the outside was the result of an inner victory in the battle between who I had been and who I was to become. Every decision about how I dressed was up for internal debate. The running commentary went something like this: *Don't you think that stripe is too bold? That sweater's a little, uh, bright, isn't it? What about that eye makeup? A bit clownish, if you ask me. And those earrings. Can't you wear something a little less . . . showy?* The thought that someone might actually start paying attention was enough to send the Fat Girl me into a panic. I was about halfway across that teetering, rickety bridge to becoming a Former Fat Girl, making my way one precarious footstep after another. The fear of what lay on the other side kept rising up, threatening to pull me back.

My first post-grad school job, in fact, was the result of one of those internal battles. After making it through the two years of classes I needed for my master's, I decided to get a job. I couldn't take being a student anymore. I was tired of being poor, of waiting for my life to begin. I was simply too impatient to stick around and finish my thesis. I'd get it done . . . sometime. So after a halfhearted search of the help-wanted ads, I was hired at a small-time restaurant-industry magazine. (Funny how I figured out a way to be around food as much as possible, isn't it?)

Before the end of my first day, I remember a little voice inside saying, "This is too easy for me." Thanks to my Fat Girl programming, I had underestimated myself yet again. I know I was lucky to be working at all back then in 1984 when jobs were scarce, but like every other kid coming out of j-school, I fantasized about being a reporter for the *New York Times* or the *Washington Post* or even the *Houston Chronicle*—a job where I could do important work, *real* work. I know there was little chance that my meager resume would end up anywhere but in the trash can at one of those major-league operations. But it didn't even occur to me to apply. I didn't have the confidence, the faith in myself, the momentum and motivation to take such a risk—not yet, anyway.

But I did have the guts to leave the campus cocoon for professional life. And I did actually *hear* that little voice that piped up on my first day. Just the fact that I heard it, that I recognized that I had aimed too low, was something of a breakthrough. Before I'd begun my Former Fat Girl journey, that little voice was buried under so many years of "I can't" that it was impossible to make out.

At the time I entered the working world, I still hadn't made any attempt to reform my eating habits. And why should I? I was big-boned, remember? My new size 8 body was the end of the line: I could go no lower, or so I thought.

Working at the restaurant magazine, I was surrounded by people who loved food, who *lived* food. The place was run by a big, bumbling fool who had a habit of laying sloppy kisses on the cheeks of the female employees every chance he got, and treated all of us "girls" in a patronizing manner that made me want to puke. The environment was so demoralizing that even those of us with the best work ethic looked for ways to slack off.

There were two good things about working at that place: the free food perks and the friends I made. Three of us formed an indelible bond in the face of our common enemy: Kim, my editor; Gabriele, the PR director; and me. We were the oppressed; the big, bad, beer-bellied boss was our oppressor. We became almost inseparable in and out of the office.

Gabriele was a fabulous cook, the closest thing I knew to a gourmet. We often ended up at her house for a meal—some elaborate feast better than anything I'd ever had at a restaurant. She was probably the first person I knew who owned a Cuisinart or at least actually used one, and she had an impressively vast culinary repertoire. She made her piecrusts from scratch (unheard of in my mom's kitchen), dabbled in exotica like tofu (*très* obscure in those days), and kept her kitchen well stocked with everything from heavy cream to saffron.

One of our standard social activities was a regular Friday night viewing of *Dallas* at Gaby's house. Gabriele would always make a feast—maybe her signature roast chicken stuffed with herbed cream cheese, cooked in a clay pot over basmati rice (my mouth is watering at the memory of it), with a fabulous tossed salad and homemade double-crust apple pie for dessert. (Notice the detail with which I describe a meal I had more than twenty years ago.)

Gaby and Kim weren't lugging around any of the Fat Girl baggage I was dealing with. Gaby was tall, maybe five feet eight and gorgeous, with olive skin, almond-shaped hazel eyes, and a wide smile. Her parents were from Germany; she was born in Canada, and her look and sense of style were European exotic to little Middle America me. She was certainly more fashion-forward than anyone I had known. And without getting too down and dirty about it, she had an enviable body— boobs just big enough (not too big) and hips just wide enough (not too wide). A real *womanly* body.

Kim was no comparison in the glamour department. She had fair skin and curly light brown hair prone to wildness. Where Gaby was voluptuous, Kim was skinny, and although I didn't think it was quite possible, she was flatter than me on top. Kim and I were more like sisters; Gaby was our captivating, sophisticated, seductive second cousin come to visit from some far-off place.

Weight wasn't much of an issue for either of them. Of course, every woman frets about a few extra pounds at least once in her life. But for Kim and Gaby, it wasn't a constant source of consternation, conflict, and internal conversation as it was for me. They basically ate what they wanted, and every once in a while, when they started to feel soft and mushy, they cracked down a bit. Neither one was into exercise really. With my almost daily running routine, *I* was the active one in the group.

It was during one of those soft and mushy moments, I

guess, that Gabriele talked Kim and me into going on the Beverly Hills Diet with her. The Beverly Hills Diet had debuted to great fanfare in the early 80s, topping the *New York Times* best-seller list for a while. For the first ten days of the diet, all you eat is fruit—different kinds of fruit on different days, but all fruit. According to Judy Mazel, the Hollywood actress who devised the plan, certain fruits have special properties. Papaya softens body fat; pineapple magically burns it off; watermelon flushes it out of your body. Huh. Who knew?

While the concept sounds complicated—not to mention utterly ridiculous—the actual plan was pretty simple. Day 1: Eat at least two pineapples, then two bananas as your last meal. Day 2: Papaya, with mango as your last meal. Some days you eat only grapes; other days, prunes; other days, watermelon. On Day 11 you get to have a half pound of bread, two tablespoons of butter, and three ears of corn, which I guess would be a treat after a week and a half of grazing in the produce section. There were no numbers to crunch, no calorie counting, no food diaries . . . and no choices. Call it enforced portion control with a dash of food group elimination, the basic tenets of many diets. Hey, it could have been worse. At least I got a good dose of fiber and some vitamins in the process.

If you've ever overdone it on grapes—the little things can be as addictive as popcorn—you know what happens. First the cramps, then the gas, and then the race to the bathroom. Imagine day after day of grapes and other fruit equally as challenging to the gastrointestinal system. When I wasn't sitting at my desk in pain, struggling to hold in the odiferous effects of the day's menu, I was in the bathroom. We all were. It was *nasty*.

For the record: I am not endorsing this diet or any diet that is basically akin to OD'ing on laxatives. I was so weak that I felt kind of drunk all the time. I couldn't think straight, and I barely had enough energy to make it through the workday. The only running I had the strength to do was to the bathroom. But I did lose weight, a lot of weight—maybe 10 pounds in the week I managed to keep up this insane regimen. (Alas, I never made it to bread, butter, and corn day.) And I couldn't believe what I saw in the mirror.

The big-boned girl I thought I was wasn't big boned at all. I had muscles. They were really there. I could see them—a little ripple in my biceps, a little definition in my thighs. For the first time since I was, I don't know, three, I could put my hand around my wrist and touch index finger to thumb. I got a glimpse of my true shape, the shape that had been hidden under layers of fat all these years.

Looking at my newly slimmer self in the mirror, I realized I wasn't finished. I had more weight to lose and more to learn about my body and myself. That vision was both a revelation and a challenge. Now I could see the finish line. I knew what winning looked like. I had to keep going.

I gained every bit of the weight back once I started eating from the rest of the food groups again, but I was no longer content with my size 8 life. Because of that diet, as crazy and unpleasant as it might have been, everything I believed about my body—my entire self-image, really—was suddenly in question. If I wasn't big boned as I'd always thought, then maybe I wasn't destined to be always the friend, never the girlfriend. Maybe I *did* have just as much of a shot at working at a major magazine or a big-time newspaper as anyone else. Maybe I *did* have a joke worth telling, an opinion worth sharing. Maybe I *could* be something other than a Fat Girl after all.

That whacked-out Beverly Hills Diet not only showed me

where the finish line was when I thought the race was over, but it made me reexamine the way I had seen myself for most of my life. I began to question the way I defined myself, the assumptions I had made about who I was and what I was capable of. I began to recognize the Fat Girl programming that had duped me into thinking I wasn't worthy, wasn't strong enough, wasn't smart enough, wasn't whatever. I began to see that the walls surrounding my comfort zone weren't made of stone at all; they were mere clouds and air. *They* weren't holding me back; *I* was holding me back.

I knew what it would take to break through: a major diet makeover. Exercise could get me only so far; I had to do something to stem my appetite. No more food free-for-alls at Gaby's house; no more mid-morning bagel runs; no more anything-goes dinners out.

I hated the thought of giving up my first love, food, even if it was standing between me and the life I wanted. The thought of going back there—to dieting, to denial, to fighting against my appetite—was downright depressing. I had reached such a positive place. My self-esteem was continuing to build little by little, and thanks to Kim and Gaby, my social life was on the upswing, too. My job was a dead end and my love life was nonexistent, but, then, you can't have it all—at least not all at once, right?

It took a full six months after that prescient experience with the Beverly Hills Diet before I decided to join Weight Watchers. I was willing to risk everything that was going right in my life for a grab at the brass ring. That's how powerful my vision was. I had gotten a glimpse of my future as a Former Fat Girl, and I wanted that life to be mine for good.

Picture Yourself as a Former Fat Girl

If you drill down to what's really so hard about losing weight, it's believing that you *can*. That's harder than passing up a platter of chocolate chip cookies warm from the oven, harder than settling into a comfy movie theater chair without the requisite tub of popcorn, harder than wrenching yourself out of bed on a winter morning to go for a workout. You're so used to thinking of yourself as a Fat Girl that it's hard to think it's possible to be anything but. And that's true whether you've had a weight issue all your life, put on pounds gradually over the years, or had a baby or two and never managed to get your prepregnancy body back. It's like those extra pounds seep into your consciousness, warping your sense of self. Being a Fat Girl—with all the thoughts and behaviors that go along with it—becomes status quo.

To begin to reverse that way of thinking, you have to find a way to feed yourself "I can" messages as often as possible. That's one of the reasons I advocate starting with exercise—to get you believing in yourself as a strong and powerful woman who can go after what you want and get it, not a prisoner of the couch, a victim of your appetite.

But that is not enough. To get to your ultimate goal— Former Fat Girlhood—you need to have a clear picture of what you're working for. You need a kind of "coming attractions" trailer for the movie of your life as a Former Fat Girl. How can you commit to chasing some nebulous new life when you don't know what that life will be? That's like agreeing to marry a guy you've never met or running a race without knowing whether the finish line is at three miles or six, or twenty-six.

You also need to tear down some of the assumptions you have about yourself. If you don't know what I'm talking about, don't worry. I didn't know what my assumptions were, either, until that drastic diet opened my eyes. I accepted as fact, for instance, that I was big boned, that I couldn't control my appetite, that I didn't belong in the "cool" crowd, that I wasn't smart enough to get into a top-tier school or talented enough to go for a high-power job, and that the guys were always more interested in my friends than they were in me.

But those things are all Fat Girl fallacies. They are not fact unless you make them so—which means that you have the power to change them, erase them, rewrite them.

A preview of the new you, the Former Fat Girl you, will help you get a giant step closer—not that I recommend you do it my way. Going on some flaky diet without medical supervision is *not* one of my Former Fat Girl Fixes, but there are tricks and tips that will, at this point in your journey, give you the kick in the pants I got when I spent a week on a fruit feeding frenzy.

You need to know where your finish line is, and that's not just some number on a scale. It's the way you want to feel physically and emotionally. It's the way you want to relate to the people around you and respond to the situations you encounter. How can you give shape to your future as a Former Fat Girl? You don't have to have a crystal ball or a standing appointment with a psychic. All you need are my fixes.

The Obstacle: Envisioning a Slimmer, Trimmer You When What You See in the Mirror Is Anything But

I know how it is: Your mind has no problem imagining all kinds of potential problems, negative consequences, and future failures, but when it comes to picturing something positive, you draw a blank. That's your Fat Girl programming at work. To short-circuit it, try these tricks.

Former Fat Girl Fixes

Keep your "skinny clothes" in your sights.

I know it's tempting to banish the little black dress you outgrew to the back of the closet (if not burn it), but you know what they say, "Out of sight, out of mind." A key piece from your "skinny" wardrobe can be a powerful visual reminder of the size you were once and could be again. If you don't have an item that would work, you have a couple of options: Cut out an inspiring picture from a magazine or catalog; download an option from a Web site; or take the ultimate risk and buy something in your goal size. You might have heard this advice before and maybe even tried it. I'm only restating it here because I found that my skinny clothes were the best check on my weight during my journey toward becoming a Former Fat Girl. I did figure out how to use the scale somewhat effectively (I'll explain how in an upcoming chapter), but being able to wear a pair of pants I hadn't been able to squeeze into in forever was more real to me than hitting some arbitrary number.

Search for role models.

Nowadays you can't touch the remote without stumbling onto some kind of makeover show. I feel like I need a shower after watching some of them, particularly the ones where some twenty-something kid is putting herself through major surgeries because she wants to look like Pamela Anderson. It's just depressing when the woman getting lipo is already a size 4. So for future Former Fat Girls' sake, flip right by those.

Some makeover shows, though, can give you a powerful dose of inspiration. One of my favorites, *The Biggest Loser*, follows seemingly normal women (and men) as they compete to see who will lose the most weight during the course of the show. You see people like you who are sincerely struggling and week after week are actually changing their bodies, their self-image, and their lives inch by inch. And it isn't all pretty, which is what makes it so inspiring. You get to see these women and men fight the same difficulties and pain you're facing. You can even see them puke (if you really want to) after a grueling workout. Watch how they change not only physically but in the way they talk about themselves and start caring more about primping and pampering. Watch as they grow to like and respect themselves in a way they didn't on the series premiere. And know this: That could be you. Sure, they're competing to win $250,000; sure, they have the pressure of knowing millions of people are watching them; sure, they have trainers and nutritionists. All of those things have to make a difference in their motivation, but resist the urge to dismiss them with "I could do it, too, if I was looking at winning a quarter of a million bucks." I'll bet that even the contestants who don't win the ultimate prize walk away with something just as valuable: a new image of themselves, a sense of self-control, and a stockpile of self-confidence that they didn't have before.

Magazines, too, can be great sources of stories about women who have shed their Fat Girl self-image (my particular favorite is *People*'s Half Their Size issue). Picture your face on their before and after shots. And note the nonphysical payoffs, how energized, confident, and sexy they feel. Remember that being a Former Fat Girl is as much about the transformation inside as it is about dropping dress sizes.

Dial back to the future.

Think about it: Was there a time in your life when you were thinner, fitter, and more confident? If so, try to re-create what your days were like then. Did you wake up happy? Did you look forward to work, school, parties, trips? Was your life bigger and busier? Were you more in demand? Did you laugh out loud?

Don't go getting all wistful on me; that's not what this little trip down memory lane is for. It is meant to inspire you, to reconnect you with the way you felt when you were at your best physically and emotionally. Try using old photo albums, videos, journals, and diaries (if you still have them) to bring that person back to life. You might even want to pull out little reminders to keep you motivated. Post a photo or two; clip a couple of quotes and put them on your computer monitor, bulletin board, or refrigerator; reread a letter from a friend that really made you feel good about yourself. These little things can keep you mindful of what you're working toward and make your goal more real for you.

Take a look at the family tree.

Some of you will say that you've never been the life of the party and never looked and felt great in a pair of jeans—that you were a Fat Girl from day one. I know it's harder for you to believe that you can overcome a whole lifetime of plus-size shopping and Fat Girl slurs. Obviously, the back-to-the-future fix won't work for you. But you know how you can often see echoes of physical characteristics among relatives, even distant ones? Try using that to your advantage. Look through your family albums to find a cousin, aunt, or grandmother with a similar body type. Try to find photos of her at her best weight. That can give you a physical point of reference to keep you motivated.

Create a virtual you.

I'm not the most technologically savvy person around, but I do know a couple of ways to use a computer to preview the new you. One option is to co-opt a tool like LandsEnd.com's My Virtual Model. You're supposed to use it to create a kind of stunt double who will "try on" clothes to see how they would look on your body (presumably as a way of finding out that the jeans you chose are cut impossibly low *before* you pay to have them shipped to you). All you do is enter your height, weight, and measurements, and up pops a computerized clone of you. To get a glimpse of you as a Former Fat Girl, create one version that reflects your body now and then take a few inches off here and there. *Voilà!* A mini you.

Another way to do it is to use a digital photo manipulation program like iPhoto or Photoshop to resize yourself. I'm not skilled enough to take on such a project myself, but I know it can be done. There's even a digital camera with an "insta-slim" feature that takes 10 pounds off with a click of a button (if only it were that easy). You could also take the low-tech route and paste a photo of your head on someone else's body. Who cares if it's silly? Whatever it takes!

Fast—the smart way.

I know what you're thinking: Is there really such a thing, a sensible way to fast? Isn't that an oxymoron like "smart bomb" or "sensitive guy"?

I'm tiptoeing into dangerous territory here, but I submit that certain types of fasts can be done safely. Simple fasting—

eating nothing and drinking only water—is not one of them. But what's called a modified fast, where you eat fruit and/or vegetables and drink fruit and vegetable juices, can be safe if you limit it to no more than three days, consult a doctor, and have no preexisting health issues (diabetes, heart disease, kidney or liver problems, for instance). You will feel weak and maybe dizzy, and you may suffer from diarrhea and the embarrassment of audible and odiferous gas, so plan the fast around any physically or socially demanding activities.

Any weight you lose during that time is water weight, and you will gain it all back, like I did. But you may also gain two things: that vision of yourself as a thinner person and a sense of control over your body that you might not think you have right now. Just being able to stick to a fruit and vegetable juice fast for one day is a willpower workout that could end up strengthening you in the long run.

If you are tempted to fast any longer than three days, this should give you pause: Prolonged fasting actually makes it harder for your body to lose weight. When it's not getting enough calories to get by, your body dials down your metabolism in an effort to conserve energy. So when you go back to eating more normally, your body will likely burn calories at a slower rate—not exactly the desired outcome.

The Obstacle: A Body That's Destined to Fail Because of Age, Pregnancies, or Less-Than-Perfect Proportions

So you don't have a supermodel inside you just waiting for her turn on the runway. Few women do. But don't let that or an aging metabolism or baby weight keep you from reaching for that Former Fat Girl life. Here's how to keep your eyes on the real prize and how not to get hung up on the myths that can keep you from grabbing it.

Former Fat Girl Fixes

Focus on your attitude, not your age.

Can you expect to regain the body of an adolescent girl if you're ten, twenty, thirty, or fifty years older? Not likely. The fact is, every woman's body loses muscle beginning in the early to mid-thirties. That contributes to a drop in metabolism of as much as 5 percent per decade after age thirty, which means that by age thirty-five you're burning about 75 fewer calories per day than you did when you were twenty-five. That means you stand to gain an extra eight pounds a year if you don't do anything to prevent it. Let me repeat: *if you don't do anything to prevent it.* Which means that *you can.* A number of researchers have shown that reasonable, regular workouts can undo, slow down, or stave off the age-related muscle loss and fat gain that could threaten your quest for Former Fat Girldom. Weight training is a particularly powerful antidote. It has even helped women in nursing homes take decades off their bodies by building muscle and bone (another thing that declines with age). The next time you're tempted to whine about being too old to change your life, just think about those iron-pumping grannies.

Chances are that it's the age in your head and not your physical age that's holding you back. We get so cynical, so jaded, don't we? With every year that passes and every life stage you blow by, it becomes harder to believe that you can make any kind of change without a whole lot of pain. You get used to driving a particular way to work, arranging your underwear drawers just so, loading the dishwasher so that all the plates lean the same way, like soldiers in formation. Any little deviation from the plan rocks your world. So why would you want to mess it all up by actually trying to be happy?

The other thing is, you're too wise for your own good now. Your faith in yourself, in other people, and in the world has been chipped away by disappointments. You aren't as ready to believe that the guy will call, the sun will shine, or the check is in the mail. You just aren't that naïve anymore. But don't use age as an excuse for not believing. If you look around, there are plenty of people who have coped and changed and reached and achieved despite the odds against them—like, uh, me.

Don't blame baby.

If you have ever been pregnant, you've experienced the curious tendency of just about everyone to tell you horror stories about botched births, hellish hospital experiences, nightmare nurses—you name it. You probably also heard that your hips, abs, butt, boobs, and basically your entire body would "never be the same." There is some truth to that. Frankly, I can't see how my body could ever be the same after squeezing an 8-pound 6-ounce person out of such a tiny place.

Pregnancy affects all women differently, but there are some universal truths about the physical aftermath: saggy breasts (that is, if you had any to start out with; I was spared this result), stretch marks, and spider veins. The ligaments holding the pelvic girdle soften while you're pregnant, sometimes leaving a pooch where you didn't have one before. Studies show that most women carry an extra five unwanted pounds into their next pregnancy. But nowhere does it say that weight gain is physically predestined. There is no law of the universe that says you can never get back to your pre-baby weight. If you tell yourself that often enough, it will be true. All you're doing is adding that to the list of assumptions you're carrying around.

Most likely, the logistics of your life as a mom are keeping you from getting your weight where you want it to be, not some pregnancy-induced metabolic glitch. Whether you are home with the kids or working in an office, you're probably . . . stressed out (strike 1), surrounded by kid-friendly snacks (strike 2), and have no time to yourself (strike 3).

I know this little revelation doesn't make it any easier for you to lose the weight, and I sympathize, I really do. But as long as you think your status as a Fat Girl is out of your control, that it's merely a physical condition, you won't be able to do anything about it. After all, I'm right there with you. As I write this, my son, Johnny, is a couple of weeks away from his fifth birthday, which means that not only am I dealing with the usual stuff—trying to keep the dust bunnies from taking over our house, making sure there's something edible for dinner tonight, helping him remember that *r* sounds like *errrr* and not *wuh* (which is kind of how he says it), and, oh yeah, working a full-time job—but I am facing the prospect of having a chunk of leftover birthday cake in my kitchen.

I gained about 42 pounds with Johnny. Breastfeeding didn't make the weight melt off magically, like it does for some people. I was a bit lactationally challenged, so that might have been it, or it could have been my hormones (I swear I looked bigger after I had Johnny than I did when I was pregnant). No, I had to work at it, and I had to make it work in this chaotic new world of mommyhood.

And it is possible. After a little more than a year, I was back in pre-baby shape without having sacrificed time with my fam-

Define the Future You

Whether you know it or not, you tell yourself all kinds of stories about who you are and how you act. To become a Former Fat Girl you have to rewrite those stories and create a new character for yourself. But you don't have to have the skills of a playwright or a novelist to do that. This exercise will get you started.

Step 1: Think about how you relate to other people and how you operate in the world—at work, at play, in love, and in your family. Then, using the numbered list under Step 1 below, complete this sentence: "I'm the kind of person who . . ." For instance, back in the day, mine would have included stuff like: "I'm the kind of person who is always the friend, never the girlfriend" and "who always puts other people's needs in front of her own" and "who hates being the center of attention" and "who never initiates conversations with strangers (especially single, available, good-looking men)." This was the box I had constructed for myself; it was the context in which I lived. Can you see how it kept me stuck in my old Fat Girl routine?

I'll bet your assumptions are pretty similar. Try to come up with at least ten. If ten is supereasy, add five more. I want you to dig deep. This is an opportunity for you to tap into that Fat Girl programming that has been controlling you for so long. You have to be able to name it before you can do anything about it.

Step 2: Here's where psychic powers will come in handy. Take a stab at another list, but this time think of how you would—excuse me, how you *will*—operate as a Former Fat Girl. Try revising the ten on your Step 1 list, and add any others that come to mind. Some of my own examples include "I'm the kind of person who doesn't let anything get in the way of my priorities (within reason)" and "who isn't afraid to voice an unpopular opinion" and "who knows how to take a compliment."

I know this is a tough exercise. If you're having trouble, think of someone whose spunk you admire, who represents some of the characteristics you want to display. That might clear your vision to make your wish list come easier.

Step 3: Review your list regularly. Add to it or change it as you discover other things about yourself on your Former Fat Girl journey. And use it as a benchmark to let you know where you are in your process because this list is one of the tools—along with the skinny clothes, the virtual you, and the other visual cues—that represent your Former Fat Girl finish line.

Step 1: You, Now "I'm the kind of person who . . ."	Step 2: Former Fat Girl "I'm the kind of person who . . ."
1:	1:
2:	2:
3:	3:
4:	4:
5:	5:
6:	6:
7:	7:
8:	8:
9:	9:
10:	10:

ily or jeopardizing my job. I was forty when I had him, so it wasn't as if I was dealing with the metabolism of a twenty-year-old. (In chapter 6 I'll tell you how to deal with the time pressures that only a mom can appreciate, how to keep your fingers out of the Goldfish and Oreos, and how to manage to do this for you when it seems as if your life is all about *them*. So stay tuned.)

Remember, the goal is not perfection.

If you asked five different women which celebrity has the "perfect" body, chances are you'd get five different answers. The point is, there's no such thing. So if you are chasing perfection, how do you know when you get there?

I know my body is not perfect. My chest is flat, my hips are wide, and my legs are big—with muscles now, not flab, but big nonetheless. I have stretch marks on my hips, and not from having a baby. There are still certain styles I can't wear, like clingy knit dresses (there's not much except hips and thighs to cling to). But this is the best body I'll ever have unless I go the surgery route, and that's not going to happen. "Easy for you to say, Ms. Size 2," you're thinking. Don't get me wrong: I'm not trying to rub it in. All I'm saying is that the way I feel matters more than the size I wear or how close I come to some idea of perfection. I have the confidence and courage to go for what I want in life; to speak, knowing that I could say the wrong thing; to reach beyond my limits, knowing that I could fall. I don't let the chance that I might fail stop me.

So when you start thinking, "My body's too old" or "My abs are shot from too many babies" or "My proportions are all off; I'm just not built that way," remember this: A Former Fat Girl isn't defined by her measurements. There isn't some qualifying weight you have to reach to be part of the club. You

know you're in when you stop letting the Fat Girl programming direct your life. You know you're in when you, too,
have the confidence to live life on your own terms. When you
are chasing a feeling and not some nebulous idea of the perfect
body, you'll know you have arrived.

After all, Secret #4 is about how to see the *whole* Former
Fat Girl you, not just get an idea of how you might look on the
outside. It's about imagining yourself going from wherever
you are now emotionally *and* physically to where you want to
be. For me, it was about seeing myself as a powerful, confident
woman who was not afraid to take a risk, whether that was
striking up a conversation with a guy or sending off my resume
for an impossible job. Secret #4 forces you to confront the
hidden assumptions about who you are and how you relate to
the world, and it gives you a clear idea of where you want to
go and what success will look and feel like. Read on for Secret
#5, a powerful tool to help you get there. Its fixes will trans-
form your relationship with food, a relationship that's hardwired into your Fat Girl programming.

Chapter Five

Secret #5: Remember, You Are Not Like Other People

When I finally started getting serious about my diet, I became a complete complainer. I had gotten used to the idea that if I was exercising regularly, I could eat whatever I wanted and not gain weight, an amazing accomplishment as far as I was concerned. If someone brought a box of doughnuts into work, how could I turn them down—even if I had already eaten a trough of cereal for breakfast? I was only being polite.

I would try to resist, but my obsession was so powerful that it wouldn't be denied. It was an itch that I just had to scratch, a flashback to childhood cases of poison ivy that burned until I just couldn't take it anymore.

Determined not to give into temptation, I would saunter

by the break room, struggling to keep from looking in the direction of the Dunkin' Donuts box on the table. I would return to my desk and try to focus on my to-do list, but all I could think about were those pillowy orbs of sugar-coated goodness. After a few futile minutes of trying to stave off the inevitable, I'd nonchalantly wander back into the break room, hoping to find the objects of my desire alone. I'd start by innocently scraping a smear of glaze from the box with my finger, telling myself that I would stop there, that I would walk away, that all I needed was a taste to satisfy me. But all that did was make me want more. "Okay" I'd tell myself, "I'll only have a half." I was only fooling myself. Half would always lead to a whole and leave me with a case of guilt worthy of a day-after adulteress.

So you can understand the problem when I joined Weight Watchers and had to come clean about every morsel I put in my mouth. Why Weight Watchers? Well, it wasn't as if my decision was the result of any kind of serious analysis of diet programs. I really didn't know anything about the Weight Watchers plan except that you ate real food, as opposed to slurping shakes or choking down prefab dinners, and that you were supposed to show up at some weekly rah-rah meeting. More important than the details of the program was what signing that check to Weight Watchers symbolized. For the first time I made a real commitment to breaking out of that Fat Girl mode I had lived in for so long. Somehow, deep inside, I knew I needed more than just a diet book or a vow to skip dessert to propel me to my future as a Former Fat Girl. I needed something more formal: a contract with my name on the dotted line. That's what Weight Watchers was to me.

Even though I thought I was ready to leave my Fat Girl past behind, Weight Watchers would be no picnic. The program forced me to become some kind of culinary accountant, a bean counter in the most literal sense. Every fingerful of frosting, every nibble of a french fry, and every shard of potato chip no matter how small factored toward my daily quota. In those days WW gave you a kind of "budget" of a certain number of servings per food group—starches, dairy, proteins, veggies, and fruits. Throughout the day you'd deduct what you ate from that budget until you had a balance of zero. No deficit spending allowed. (Maybe we should get Congress in on that action.)

WW had strict specifications for what constituted a serving. A "bowlful" or a "hamburger patty" or a "pizza slice" wasn't enough. How big was the bowl? How much did the burger weigh? What were the exact dimensions of the pizza slice and the cheese-to-crust-to-sauce ratio?

You know I was no stranger to dieting, but this took calorie conservation to a whole new level. I had to buy a tiny scale to weigh my cereal, use a cup measure to parcel out my measly portion of sliced strawberries, and pull out a ruler to calculate the precise size of the cheese slice I was preparing for my afternoon snack. I felt like one of those science geeks on *CSI:*, as though my kitchen had become a lab where I was constantly dissecting my diet, parsing out nutrients so I could match my meals to the Weight Watchers specs. This was back in the old days, before you could simply key the components of your meal into your Treo or laptop and have it magically calculated for you. It is still the same attention to detail but with a lot less hassle.

I felt like I was suffocating under all these rules, rules, rules. I resented sacrificing the freedom to indulge my appetite. I was used to grazing in open fields without any real restrictions; now this damn diet was fencing me in, cutting me off from the foods I loved before I had eaten my fill. I literally mourned the absence of my food faves, especially carbs—pasta, rolls, biscuits, you name it. It wasn't like my beloved starches were completely verboten, but the drastically downsized WW portions were just a tease. Anything less than my usual plate of spaghetti the size of a Hummer hubcap, and I was miserable. And I let everyone around me know it.

Nevertheless, I dutifully abided by the WW guidelines, but not without a whole lot of kvetching and obtrusive stomach growling. I felt like I was more obsessed with food than ever. I had to plan everything I ate down to the tiniest morsel, to calculate the impact of each nibble on the day's bottom line. There was no longer such a thing as a casual bite; everything I put into my mouth was intentional.

I started bringing my lunch to work to avoid having to navigate restaurant menus for WW-appropriate meals (and the temptation of blowing an entire day's quota by noon). Lunch consisted of a turkey and low-fat cheese sandwich on low-cal bread and carrot sticks. Now remember, this was before there were entire aisles of reduced-fat and fat-free foods. There was no low-fat mayonnaise. There were no Baked Lays or cheddar soy crisps to sub for a bag of greasy chips. The light bread wasn't bad except that it was so airy you could practically read a newspaper through it. Cheese was another story. Its texture was not unlike the paste that we used to make crafts in elementary school, and the taste wasn't far off, either (and I'm speaking from experience). It was nothing like the low-fat cheeses you can get today that are almost identical to the real thing.

As unsatisfying as my main dish might have been, I tried to eat it as slowly as I could, struggling to make it and the bag of carrots last the entire lunch hour. If I ended fifteen minutes short, I would spend those fifteen minutes thinking about what I *could* be eating or how long it would be until dinner when I could eat again.

Compared to the sandwich, the carrots were a treat. Raw carrots were practically the only vegetable other than potatoes and corn that I actually liked at the time. I couldn't stand them cooked to an orangey mush; but raw, they had a nice crunch and a subtle sweetness. And on WW, back in the day, they were a "free" food, meaning they could be eaten in unlimited quantities. (I love the phrase *unlimited quantities*.) Since veggies were the only thing I could let loose on, they became my staple. I started eating carrots the way I used to eat popcorn (see *unlimited quantities* reference above). They became my snack of choice, anytime, anywhere.

After several months of feeding my carrot habit, something curious happened: I started turning orange. A friend noticed it first, catching a glimpse of my palms that looked a bit like they were stained from a bad self-tanner. The color soon spread to my arms, feet, legs, and face. I didn't really see it, but other people did. I guess I had just gotten used to the look. One friend grew so alarmed that she looked it up in a medical text (remember, this was before Google). Diagnosis: beta-carotene overload. Common in vegetarians and infants who OD'd on pureed carrots and sweet potatoes, in extreme circumstances too much of this form of vitamin A can lead to brain damage, or so they say. I certainly haven't seen any evidence of that in myself, unless you count short-term memory loss ("Now, what did I come in here for?"), long-term memory loss ("What do you mean I was born in Kentucky?"), and lack of mental focus (I was going to give you an example, but I got caught up staring out the window at nothing in particular).

Seriously, all is well. I curbed my carrot obsession a bit,

substituting celery, which held no similar risks but wasn't as exciting (not that carrots were exactly thrilling, either, but you know what I mean). The whole experience became something of a joke among my friends, so much so that I dressed as a carrot for a Halloween party one year. I was orange from the neck down, my face was green, and my equally as green hair was spiked like a punk rocker to simulate the stem and leaves.

If that getup doesn't prove how far I had come in my whole social development cycle, I don't know what will. Little old wallflower me, dressed for Halloween not as a ghost or hobo or something equally as nondescript, but as a neon orange, look-at-me-I'm-on-display carrot. Little old hermit me with a party on her calendar—one that doesn't involve family members. Little old misfit me with friends to call her own and not imaginary ones.

I was continuing to work the Former Fat Girl program. I was still running, feeling better and stronger after every day on the trail. Plus, I was making other kinds of strides. Soon after dabbling in the Beverly Hills Diet, Kim, Gabriele, and I vowed to get new jobs and get out of our workplace hell. We made a bet: Whichever of us got a job first won a fabulous lunch at the place of her choice, courtesy of the other two. With a prize like lunch, there was no competition. I had to win.

And I did. I landed a job at the weekly business newspaper in Austin. It was no *Wall Street Journal*, but it was a teeny step up from what I had been doing. It also said something for my self-esteem to make the break from my beer-bellied boss and his prison rule. (Lunch, in case you're interested, was at The Four Seasons. Delish, as my nana used to say.) I was at the business journal when I joined Weight Watchers.

In the meantime, I had started going to a new church with a cool pastor and a small but active group of twenty-somethings.

I had found the church through a friend from college who was working there as the youth minister. I was drawn to the no-nonsense, real-life way that Father Jordan spoke to us at Mass. I was drawn to the energy that the young adults group seemed to have as I sized them up over the first couple of months after I started attending services there. They were a very social crowd; it wasn't all Bible study and prayer meetings. (We're talking about Catholics, remember.) They had happy hours, Super Bowl parties, after-Mass brunches, all kinds of stuff. There were people from all over, transplants to Austin during the tech boom of the mid to late 80s: Eddie from Cleveland, a loud guy with a kidlike sense of humor who wore his passion for his hometown on his sleeve; Maureen from somewhere in the Midwest who told sweet, funny stories about her special ed students; and John, a New Yorker whose know-it-all tendencies could get a bit obnoxious but who was one of the quirky characters that made the group fun.

Slowly, slowly, I started getting involved. I went to a Mass at one of the group members' homes and chatted over dinner afterward. I helped with a fund-raiser for a sister church in a poor central Texas town. I showed up at one of those happy hours and then another and another. Someone talked me into signing up for the group's volleyball team. Ten years after I had flunked tryouts in tenth grade, there I was, serving and setting (I was too short to spike) on a shiny wooden court.

The interesting thing was, these people—like Kim and Gabriele—didn't know the old Fat Girl me. They only knew the size 8 me standing in front of them. They knew me as a runner, as an athlete, even! They didn't know how socially inept I had been, how terrified the old Fat Girl would have been at the idea of showing up in a pair of shorts to run around and sweat with *boys*.

I was again establishing my identity with a new group of people, much like I had done as a freshman in college. But I wasn't the Fat Girl I used to be; no, far from it. I found myself taking chances with this new group as never before: dancing by myself, laughing out loud, and courting attention (at least a little). I was inching my way out of the dark anonymity of the wings and closer to center stage, and it was scary—but I liked it. I liked it enough to keep going.

All of those good things—the new job, the new friends, the revenge of the nerd on the volleyball court—made me want even more what Weight Watchers was offering: a chance to become even more of myself, to truly become comfortable in my own skin. Even so, I had moments when my mouth watered for a late-night burger and beer with the softball team, when I was dying for an order of pancakes at brunch after church instead of the scrambled eggs and dry wheat toast on my plate.

It would take an offhand comment from a fed-up friend to jolt me out of my self-pity and into a new attitude about the whole Weight Watchers thing. It happened one day after I had finished counting out a paltry pile of Wheat Thins to accompany a postage-stamp-size cube of cheddar. "Why do I have to think about food all the time?" I bitched to my friend Kim. "Why can't I eat like other people?"

I didn't really expect an answer, but I got one. Kim looked at me and said in her matter-of-fact way, "Because, Lisa, you are not like other people."

Now that, Oprah fans, was an aha! moment.

I know Kim didn't realize she was saying anything particularly insightful. She was probably so sick of my bellyaching (how's that for a play on words?) that she was just trying to shut me up. And she did. That statement was so right, so brilliant, so straight to the heart of the matter that I was speechless.

You are not like other people. Of course I'm not! I realized that those good old days I yearned for when I supposedly ate what I wanted without a second thought were only an illusion. In reality, I had never taken food lightly. I had never been able to think about food without conjuring up all sorts of emotions. From the outside I might have looked as though I just didn't care when I went back to the dessert buffet for seconds, but inside there was a world-class battle going on. My insatiable desire for food and lack of control over my appetite made me feel worthless, insecure, and inadequate. In the face of temptation, I felt weak, hopelessly weak. Oh, and the guilt; can't forget that one. It was like I was born with a physiological response: As soon as I started to chew, the Fat Girl feelings began to flow.

I had spent years envying people whose lives didn't revolve around food, who could eat with true abandon. I used to watch in awe as they indulged unselfconsciously, wondering what it would be like to be able to do that. Wondering if I'd ever be able to take a bite of something that wasn't on the official list of diet foods (celery sticks, saltine crackers, skinless chicken breasts—you know them by heart) and not hear a voice in my head ask, "Do you really think you should?"

My mistake was in thinking that silencing that voice would be as easy as switching off an annoying talk radio show. But as I thought about what Kim said, I began to realize that, at least for me, it wouldn't be easy. It *couldn't* be easy. I had all those Fat Girl feelings to deal with. It wasn't like I could hit some "off" button and they'd disappear.

It began to make sense to me why living by some list of officially sanctioned diet foods never worked for me before, why the different weight loss gimmicks, no matter how scientifically solid, never budged the needle on the scale much. For me it was more about *how* to eat than *what* to eat. I had to make my own way; I had to take the nuggets of wisdom in my weight loss experiences of the past, toss in all those Fat Girl feelings associated with food, and frappe them together into a new Former Fat Girl formula.

Realizing that I had a unique relationship with food helped me stop comparing myself to the people around me and to accept that I had to make my own choices based on who I was. I began to be okay with the fact that while everyone else at the table was chowing down on chicken-fried steak and mashed potatoes, I was munching on a chef salad (dressing on the side, no ham, no cheese). I began to stop expecting myself to leave half of my dessert on the plate as other girls seemed to do so easily. I began to accept the fact that for me it was better not to order it in the first place, because once it was in front of me, there was no stopping. I began to define a "new normal" for myself, one that was based on a true understanding of my feelings and attitudes about food as a Fat Girl.

I knew I was different, and I also knew what I wanted. I wanted a body I could be proud of and feel truly comfortable in. But I also wanted to start treating myself well. I wanted to feed myself well, keep myself well watered, nurture myself as you do a seed that you're trying to coax into a flower. I wanted to be healthy and feel the energy and confidence that comes from living healthfully. I wanted to continue to take the kind of risks I had just started to take—meeting new people and trying new things—without letting fear or any kind of physical limitations stop me. And I knew that recognizing and dealing with my unique relationship with food would be key to getting me there.

Work with Your Differences

It might not be the easiest thing for you to embrace the whole "You are not like other people" idea. At first it could seem like a confirmation of how you've always felt—like an outsider, a misfit. I know it did for me. I had spent my whole life wanting to belong, and "You are not like other people" wasn't exactly an invitation to an exclusive party.

Deep down, though, it all makes sense. There has to be a reason that you haven't been able to stick with a diet long enough to reach your goal weight. There has to be a reason that you have to diet at all. When you think about it, diets are relatively straightforward: Strip away all the whys and wherefores, and what's left is a simple list of do's and don'ts. All that's left is for you to follow orders, right?

But because of all the emotions wrapped up in being a Fat Girl, it's way more complicated than that. For you, eating is anything but straightforward. It's more emotional than a trashy romance novel because it's so personal. You can see it, I know. You know how ashamed you feel when you vow not to overindulge and then break that vow—again. You aren't like other people. You can't casually eat what you want without an internal struggle. It takes a Herculean effort to push away your plate while there is still even the smallest morsel on it and say, "I'm full." Even though you may feel full physically, you're never really satisfied.

You need to reprogram yourself. Forget the lists of "approved" foods. It's not about that. It's about knowing how to treat yourself well, how to make better choices, how to eat less and still be satisfied, and how to eat healthfully no matter where you are or how much time you have. This kind of guidance will reshape your relationship with food in a way you can live with for the rest of your life. And that's what it means to be a Former Fat Girl. It isn't a six-week, six-month, or six-year plan. It's a new way of living.

I've done the heavy lifting for you. I've created a Former Fat Girl formula for losing weight that emphasizes the strategies and tactics that will work for you. No matter how many times you've tried before, no matter how hard this "reprogramming" sounds, you can do it. You can change that emotionally toxic relationship you have with food. I'm living proof that it's possible.

The Obstacle: You Weren't Born with an Appetite Off Switch

Well, me neither. Unfortunately, that doesn't seem to be standard equipment for Fat Girls, but here are some work-arounds that will help satisfy you without sabotaging your Former Fat Girl quest.

Former Fat Girl Fixes

Become an illusionist.

I know it feels like a rip-off when all you get is a measly tablespoon or two of mashed potatoes and you're used to heaping helpings. On some level we all eat with our eyes. The pleasure and satisfaction we get from food starts kicking in when we see it on the plate. Some people are turned on by colors and textures and the prospect of sampling something they've never tasted before, but Fat Girls are hardwired to get a kick from quantity. If your plate isn't full enough, if the fried chicken

Guide to Low- and High-Density Foods

It's simple: The lower a food falls on the density scale, the more water, air, and/or fiber it contains, and the more you can eat! Here is your guide from low to high, from nutrition researcher Barbara Rolls, Ph.D., of Pennsylvania State University.

Very Low Density: Eat with Abandon (Almost) Most veggies (except starchy ones, like potatoes), fruits (especially berries, melons, citrus fruits, and apples), fat-free dairy foods such as yogurt (unsweetened or artificially sweetened), and skim milk. Oh, yeah, and water.

Low Density: Green-Light These Foods Within Reason Cooked whole grains, like oatmeal and brown rice, breakfast cereals (watch out for the granola, though), frozen yogurt, lean meats, tofu, legumes (aka black beans, chickpeas, etc.), cottage cheese, starches like potatoes and pasta, sugary fruits like grapes, and starchy fruits like bananas.

Medium Density: Proceed with Caution Most cheeses, ice cream, dried fruits, low-fat baked goods, and such snacks as pretzels, cookies, baked chips, air-popped popcorn, whole wheat bread, bagels, English muffins, and eggs.

High Density: Tread Lightly (Because These Foods Are Not Light) Regular crackers, cookies, chocolate, frostings, nuts, butter, and full-fat condiments like mayonnaise.

Source: Adapted with permission from *Volumetrics: Feel Full on Fewer Calories* by Barbara Rolls and Robert A. Barnett (HarperCollins, 2000).

breast isn't big enough (or as big as the one on the next person's plate), you immediately start thinking you're going to need more. And you start figuring out a way to get it even before the first bite touches your lips. How can you expect to know when you've eaten enough to be sated if you already have it in your head that you won't be?

There are ways, I've discovered, to fulfill your desire for quantity or at least trick yourself into thinking you're eating more than you are. The first is to create the illusion of substance by focusing on foods that have a lot of water, air, or fiber in them. Because they're bloated with those noncaloric elements, you can have larger portions of these foods without blowing your calorie quota. You won't find Godiva chocolate on the list or Gorgonzola cheese or penne pasta. The foods with the lowest calorie density are primarily vegetables (excluding starchy ones like potatoes) and puffy cereals (like Rice Krispies), not exactly what you'd request at your last meal. (See the sidebar above for more examples.) This little tactic helped me when I was weighing and measuring everything. I found out quickly, for instance, that low-fat granola was a really bad choice for breakfast. It was so heavy that I could have only a couple of spoonfuls; for the same number of calories I could have almost five times as much Bran Chex. That sure made a difference in my attitude toward the diet by short-circuiting that ripped-off feeling.

Here are a couple of other illusions to try: Use a salad plate instead of a dinner plate so that your meal doesn't look so sparse. Research shows that dinner plates have increased in size over the past several years, almost to the size of a meat platter. The bigger the plate, the smaller a normal-size portion looks—and the more likely you will feel cheated and want more. Also, try using salad forks and teaspoons instead of dinner forks and soup spoons (I'm expecting a hand slap from Ms. Manners for this). If you haven't noticed, eating utensils have been super-sized, too.

Take it slow.

Using smaller utensils doesn't just fool you into thinking you're taking in a more substantial bite, it also slows the whole meal down for the simple reason that you can't fit as much on your fork. Eating slowly helps you get more pleasure out of food (you can actually *taste* it, for one thing), so maybe you won't need as much of it. I come from a family of speed eaters, so don't think this is an easy thing for me. But I started doing it in self-defense when I began bringing my Weight Watchers–compliant lunch to work. I did all kinds of little things to make it last; setting my sandwich down, taking a sip of water, then a bite of carrot, then another sip of water. An observer might have thought I was a bit OCD, but I was just trying to resist the urge to stuff the entire sandwich in my mouth at one time.

Another slo-mo option: Eat with chopsticks. For years I ate all my dinners at home with an Asian flair, no matter what kind of cuisine: salads, stir-fries, pasta, you name it. Of course, chopsticks are particularly effective dieting tools if you don't know how to use them; chances are, only a fraction of what you're eating will actually make it to your mouth. But even if you have expert stick skills, you'll find they make any meal more leisurely, more enjoyable, and more like a "time-out" from life versus a plate-cleaning race.

Chew your calories.

Not as in "stop swallowing your food whole" (although if that's an issue for you, consider this a cease-and-desist order). I mean cut down or cut *out* sodas, juices, teas, or other liquids that contain calories. When you are trying to limit the number of calories you're eating, it makes sense to "spend" them only on the things that will leave you the most satisfied, and it's tough to feel the full impact, flavor, and texture of a drink you're sucking down through a straw. There are scientific studies that back up the fact that liquid calories don't make as much impact on satisfaction as calories that come from solid food, but I didn't need a study to tell me that. Long before researchers came up with that conclusion, I had taught myself to savor Diet Coke—actually prefer it—and make the "real thing" an INO. There was no way I'd waste some of my precious calories on a soda, not if it meant I couldn't have something I wanted even more, like bread or a bit of pasta. Also, I know people have all kinds of problems with Splenda and other artificial sweeteners, and I'm by no means telling you to drink the stuff if you don't want to. There are other noncaloric liquid libations you can have. (Water comes to mind.) If you want something with a little flavor, you can try flat or sparkling water infused with a touch of fruit like lime or orange, like the new Hint brand drinks (www.drinkhint.com) or citrus-spiked Perrier. No sugar, no chemicals, no calories.

Speaking of fruit, while fruit juices are head-over-heels healthier than soda, they do contain lots of calories that won't make much of a dent in your appetite. It is better to eat the orange, apple, or grapefruit itself and give your choppers something to do.

Be wasteful.

It's already obvious that I don't buy into many of the mores of our society, the rules of good manners, the laws governing proper use of handicap-accessible restrooms, and so forth. And here I go again. At the risk of earning a spot on the "questionable" list for admission to the afterlife, I'm suggesting that you trash the remaining Halloween candy in your pantry before it ends up on your hips; the leftover birthday cake you made for your sister; the rest of the double-decker sub on your plate that you certainly don't need to eat and aren't even hungry for. That's right: Trash it. Throw it away. And don't just put it in the kitchen waste bin because a little thing like botulism won't stop a Fat Girl from a little Dumpster diving. I'll admit right here that I have been known to actually dig a lump of cake or a piece of candy out of the trash can in my kitchen, and I know I'm not the only one. I have a friend who douses stuff with water to ruin it before she puts it in the trash so she won't be tempted. Do whatever it takes: Foul it, put the can out at the curb to use your watchful neighbors as a deterrent, or give it to the dog next door (unless it's chocolate, which is deadly for dogs).

You could use the standard strategy of bringing leftovers to work, but that method isn't foolproof. You still have to deal with the temptation posed by a platter of tantalizing break room snacks (see previous doughnut anecdote). No, despite the fact that it goes against everything our mothers taught us, wastefulness is the way to go. After all, are you going for sainthood or Former Fat Girlhood? And if you're on a budget and this feels wasteful, think about the extra bucks you'll have to spend later on a health club membership or weight loss program.

Put your mind where your mouth is.

Really getting in touch with why you eat can help you start shutting down your appetite when it's had enough. For instance, I bet you would say you eat because you like food. It makes you feel good. It comforts you when you're sad, tired, stressed, or lonely. And I believe you. But that's not the whole story. Have you ever thought that on some level maybe you're using food to punish yourself, too? Your Fat Girl programming drives you to eat anything and everything, overriding all common sense, all vanity, all ego, all the qualities you might respect in yourself. (I have dug around for food in the *trash*, for God's sake!) Why else would you continue to eat when you know you're full, when you don't even like what you're putting in your mouth, when you know that what you're doing is unhealthy physically and emotionally? I love food. I love reading about it, trying new dishes, and discovering new recipes and techniques. I have loved food since I was a kid. But for a long time I couldn't distinguish between a healthy passion for food and an unhealthy drive to eat. I used my love of food to justify abusing myself with it. It's kind of like some women I know who refuse to stop wearing three-inch heels despite the fact that they end up in agony at the end of the day.

Okay, so where does that leave you? You need to start thinking about what you're putting in your mouth and *what's in it for you*. Think about all the good things food does for you: It satisfies your physical hunger, gives you all kinds of good nutrients, and—just as important—pampers you, treats you, pats you on the back, serves as a kind of gustatory hug. Anything you eat, whether it's an apple or a potato chip, a burger or a bonbon, can do good things for you. What matters more than how many fat grams it has or how many calories it packs is *why* you're eating it. Start asking: "What will [insert food here] do *for* me?" You'll be surprised at how many times the answer is "Nothing." Simply asking that question over and over again until it becomes a reflex (which it will) is a major first step. Soon you'll find yourself, believe it or not, walking away from the buffet table, walking away from that platter of cookies in the break room, and stopping your hand midair as you reach for a glob of icing on the cake plate.

Here's an example: Living in Texas, I ate at a lot of Mexican restaurants where they served unlimited (there's that word again) baskets of tortilla chips and salsa. I had and still have a particular fondness for chips that are folded over flat like little smushed taco shells. Because they were my favorites, I'd paw through the basket to find the folded chips (rude, I know) and eat them first. Once they were gone, I'd move on to the substandard ones, the curved ones, the flat ones, whatever. But when I started asking myself, "What will these chips do *for* me?" I figured out that the folded chips were the ones I really wanted; the rest of them were second-rate. I was eating them for the hell of it, because they were there. So I made a rule: I would eat *only* folded chips. If there happened to be five in the basket, I could eat five. If there were zero, tough luck. To this day if you go to eat Mexican food with me, you'll see me digging for those folded chips. I only pray that no one starts selling entire bags of folded chips, as they do broken pretzels and muffin tops and doughnut holes, or there might be a sequel to this book (*Former Fat Girl No More: The Great Tortilla Chip Debacle*).

The Obstacle: The Confusing, Complicated, and Ultimately Aggravating Portion Control Issue

In this land of bigger is better (with the exception of bellies, butts, and thighs), we have lost all perspective on how much a

Drink or Chew? The Caloric Costs

Drink	Chew
12-ounce Coke Classic (145 cals)	2 Nutter Butter Peanut Butter Cookies (130 cals)
16-ounce Snapple Raspberry Tea (200 cals)	1 Small McDonald's fries (210 cals)
1 can Slim Fast (220 cals)	1 slice medium Domino's cheese pizza (187 cals)
Grande Starbucks Frappuccino (247 cals)	Subway 6-inch turkey sandwich (280 cals)
12-ounce Red Bull (187 cals)	Package Reese's Peanut Butter Cups (180 cals)

Source: Food labels, product websites.

"normal" portion is. How do you downsize your expectations? Try my fixes.

Former Fat Girl Fixes

Become a label reader.

The Nutrition Facts labels on packaged foods tell you everything you need to know about what's inside, and then some. The sheer volume of data can be overwhelming, but there are a few key facts to pay attention to:

- *Serving size:* Very important. All the info on the rest of the label—the number of calories, fat grams, fiber, etc.—are keyed to the serving size. Look for this tidbit of info just under the Nutrition Facts heading.
- *Calories:* Remember that the number of calories listed in this spot relates to the specified serving size. I don't mean to nag you about this, but it can get tricky. For instance, some things that appear to be single-serving packages (such as bags of chips, muffins, and even microwavable soup) are actually meant to serve more than one. So don't make any assumptions: Check the serving size and then look at the calories. You don't want to work your way through a "Big Grab" bag of potato chips—even if they're Baked Lays—only to find out that you've eaten twice as many calories as you intended.
- *Total Fat/% of Daily Value:* The number of fat grams isn't as important as how much of your total daily fat allowance you're spending on a serving. Look for this figure in the right column just opposite the Total Fat figure. The percentage of Daily Value is based on a 2,000-calorie-per-day diet,

so you'll have to adjust down if you're trying to consume fewer calories. Checking this number will help you decide if you really want to use half of your daily allowance on a honey bun from the vending machine.

- *Saturated Fat and Trans Fat:* These fats, listed as subcategories under the Total Fat line, may contribute to heart disease. Try to keep them as low as possible. Your total daily saturated fat allowance is 20 grams, so even 4 grams is a substantial amount. Right now there is no established limit on trans fat, but dietitians suggest keeping your intake as low as possible—zero if you can manage it.

- *Fiber:* The fiber figure is hard to find on labels. It's listed as a subcategory under Total Carbohydrate. But don't miss it. Fiber can help keep you feeling fuller longer (not to mention help prevent all kinds of diseases, like heart disease and cancers), and most women don't get nearly enough. Look for cereals and breads with at least 3 grams per serving, and eat lots of veggies to make your daily quota of 25 grams.

- *Protein:* Usually at the end of the main list on labels, protein is also a great appetite satisfier. The "% of Daily Value" just opposite the number of protein grams can give you an idea of whether the item you're looking at packs a good amount of protein because it's hard to tell from the number of grams. For instance, I don't know from 16 grams of protein, but when I see that it's 32 percent of my daily quota, that sounds pretty good.

Write it down, write it *all* down.

I know you're gonna hate this one as much as I did, and I would spare you if I could. But you've got to do it. You've got to write every bite down in a little book or on your Blackberry or somewhere so you know how many calories you're eating each day. That's the only way to tell if you're taking in more than you're burning off—and that, despite other diet gurus' attempts to convince you differently, is the only scientifically proven way to lose weight. Knowing that one serving of linguine is one cup and about 200 calories or that a serving of bread is one slice (not two) will be a major reality check because you know you can't trust yourself to stop when you're full like everybody else. (Remember, *you are not like other people*.) You need to compensate for that. Asking yourself what you're getting out of each bite is a start, but knowing what that bite will cost you in terms of calories might just give you the strength to walk away. You won't have to do it forever, I promise. Eventually, you'll be able to eyeball a bowl of cereal and know exactly when to stop pouring. But until that happens, be strong. Use my guidelines on page 160 to help you size up your servings. (One trick: I used cup measures instead of serving spoons to help me keep my perspective.) Document for at least three months. If that sounds like a long time, consider this: I did it for over a year, until I felt like I could trust myself not to cheat. Even when you think you've got it down, pull out that scale or ruler and check yourself every couple of months to help stay on track.

No fat, low fat, full fat—treat all treats the same.

In most cases, low-fat and no-fat versions of treats like cookies and snack cakes pack the same number of calories as the full fat version, or only slightly fewer. Many manufacturers pump up the sugar to help distract your taste buds from the missing fat. So don't think you can eat three low-fat Chips Ahoy instead of two regular ones unless the label says differently. And if the number of calories is similar, think hard about whether you want to buy the low-fat product at all. Low fat may mean low quality (although we've come a long way from that pasty excuse for cheese that I had in the mid to late 80s). The last thing you want to do is end up stuffing yourself with some lame low-fat cookies to satisfy a craving when you could have had one or two of what you really wanted for fewer calories.

Identify your addiction and take special control measures.

I think I've said it before, at least a couple of times: I love any food whose first ingredient is flour: bread, bagels, yeast rolls, soft pretzels, pasta, pizza crust (the sauce and cheese are nice touches, but I'm really in it for the crust). My secret dream is to one day go to France and become an apprentice bread maker. I could exist completely on sesame seed bagels with a thin smear of light cream cheese and strawberry jam. Can I stop now? Do you get it? Me plus bread equals love.

I knew when I started Weight Watchers that I'd have the most trouble cutting back on my friends from the bakery. And why was that? Because it was the baked goods, beyond all other foods, that I was most likely to overeat. So after the first six weeks on the diet, when I was allowed to increase my daily allotment of bread portions from six to eight, I held steady at six. I knew I had to break my addiction to bread and force myself to play the field, to learn to enjoy the company of other consumables. And I did. I became fond of all kinds of vegetables I had previously avoided in pursuit of my passion: zucchini, yellow squash, and green and red peppers. My salads were a farmer's market menagerie of at least seven kinds of veggies. I ate broccoli every day in salads, as a topper for potatoes, or just plain steamed on the side, maybe with a little soy sauce. I still have a soft spot for bread; to this day I keep an eye on my portions, particularly of pasta and pizza.

You know what food or foods you crave. You know what your downfall is, the thing you've missed most when you've dieted in the past, the thing you turn to when you're stressed or celebrating, or just letting go. Your challenge right now is to limit what you love—not cut it out completely; that would sabotage your Former Fat Girl quest. You need to set a strict limit, a challenging limit, and stick to it. For instance, if your love is chocolate, allow yourself one small piece a day, no more. And watch what happens: First, you will begin to appreciate chocolate even more. It will become a real treat, something you look forward to and savor as never before. You'll experience its flavor and texture more intensely. It is the old absence-makes-the-heart-grow-fonder thing.

If you're cutting back drastically on a food that had been a major source of calories in your diet, you'll start to see results on the scale. So, to carry my chocolate example further, if you're used to snacking from the bowl of M&Ms on your desk all day and cut back to one pack (the 1.69-ounce size, not the half-pound bag), you'll save about 700 calories. That is nothing to sneeze at. If you bank 700 calories every day, you'll lose almost 6 pounds in one month!

Don't skip the appetizers.

You weren't expecting to hear *that*, were you? But what I mean is, order an appetizer instead of an entrée, not in addition. The reasoning: Today's appetizers are the size of yesterday's entrées, so by ordering an appetizer, you're more likely to get a reasonable portion (with the exception of appetizers meant to be shared, like mountains of nachos and fried mushrooms). And many times, especially at white tablecloth restaurants, the appetizer menus are actually more interesting than the entrées (that's the foodie in me talking). Order a small salad to start if you want and then ask the waiter to bring your appetizer selection with the entrées. I've never had a waiter turn up his or her nose at that request.

Hit the convenience store.

Don't expect to suddenly stop needing Cheetos. Changes like that take time. If you absolutely must have a bag, swing by the Stop 'n Go and get the single serving size (*not* the Big Grab). The convenience store is also the perfect place to get *one* Tootsie Roll or *one* Reese's Peanut Butter Cup the size of a quarter (look for them near the checkout) instead of a bag you'll be tempted to polish off in a couple of sittings. The convenience store makes portion control, uh, convenient. Use it.

Practice safe snacking.

It may be cheaper to buy the big box of Wheat Thins than the preportioned 100-calorie packs, but what do you want more: a bigger bank account or a smaller dress size? Stop buying in bulk just to get a bargain, thinking you'll be able to cut yourself off at one portion. Remember, you are not like other people. Remove the temptation altogether by buying preportioned snacks. In the last couple of years, food companies have smartened up to the fact that individual servings of crackers and cookies aren't just good for kids' lunch boxes; they're great for adults with calorie control issues, too. Many companies have introduced snacks such as crackers and "cookie crisps" (aka lower-fat versions of Oreos and Nutter Butters) in the individual 100-calorie size. They can help you snack smarter. Another option is to buy those tiny snack-size Ziplocs and create your own individual portions. If you think you can do that

How to Know If You're Too Obsessed

As you fight against your Fat Girl programming, be careful not to go overboard. Don't take your new healthy habits, like counting calories, weighing food, and weighing yourself, to an unhealthy extreme. These are only a few of the warning signs.

- Frequent weighing (more than once a day)
- Loss of focus at school or work
- Rituals like drinking only from a certain cup or eating certain foods on certain days (my tortilla chip fixation might have applied if I did it daily)
- Loss of menstrual periods
- Chronic fatigue or dizziness
- Taking laxatives, throwing up, or prolonged fasting
- Thinning hair

If anything on this list sounds like you, get help. A great place to start is the Renfrew Center, one of the top eating disorder clinics in the country. Its Web site (www.renfrewcenter.com) can help you with your next steps.

without slipping extra into each bag (or into your mouth), go for it.

Discover frozen dinners (if you haven't already).

Frozen dinners are great for controlling portion size, especially for working lunches at your desk, because there's not much food around to supplement your supper. The "healthy" brands, such as Lean Cuisine, Healthy Choice, and South Beach, all feature some pretty decent dishes. (I like Lean Cuisine's Asian entrées in particular.) You typically get larger portions for fewer calories than you would with a non-diet-conscious line such as Stouffer's or Amy's (which features organic foods). But read the labels for calories and fat content; some of the Stouffer's and Amy's entrées are only slightly higher than the diet lines and could be tastier and more satisfying.

Don't be afraid to obsess.

Here's the thing: You have to obsess to some extent to break out of those Fat Girl eating habits and shed the Fat Girl mindset. By obsessing I mean measuring, weighing, keeping a calorie tally. I mean using INO out the wazoo. I mean setting rules about what you will and will not eat and how much, like the weird little rule I use to keep myself from munching my way through a whole basket of tortilla chips and salsa. You will get flack for this from outside observers; I'll get into that more in the next chapter. But trust yourself, trust me, and trust the Former Fat Girl program: You have to take the hard line if you want to reach your goals physically and personally. That said, food obsessions can become disorders; there's no doubt about that. If you think you might be going over the edge, see the sidebar on page 158 to decide for sure and get help.

Sizing Things Up

A little cheat sheet for girls with portion control issues		
Food	Portion	Picture This
Bread	1 slice	a CD case
Cheese	1 ounce	4 dice
French fries	10 fries	a TV remote control
Ice cream	½ cup	a baseball
Meat (beef, poultry, etc.)	3 ounces	an Altoids box
Nuts	⅓ cup	2 C batteries
Pancake	one 4-inch pancake	a DVD
Pasta	1 cup	a tennis ball

Source: Adapted from the National Cholesterol Education Program (hin.nhlbi.nih.gov /portion).

Don't be distracted by the diet debates.

It's hard not to get caught up in the arguments over which weight loss program is best, especially because you've probably had personal experience with many. You want to believe there's another way, a better way, a gimmick that will make it easier. But here's the reality: There's always going to be something new or at least a new take on an old concept. And it's highly unlikely that any one approach—low carb, low cal, low fat, or low sugar—is going to emerge as the clear winner. Trying to follow diet trends and sort fact from fiction will only confuse you and keep you from focusing on your own journey, which is (remember?) more about how and why you eat than what you eat.

I didn't know this, either, until the day Kim dropped that little bomb on me so many years ago. I needed Secret #5 to drive home that point, to make it clear that I had issues with food that other people didn't have and that expecting myself to find some cookie-cutter diet that would take the weight off for good was just an exercise in frustration. Secret #5 helped me— and will help you—zero in on the particular challenges of losing weight when you have Fat Girl baggage and figure out how to deal with it.

But as you begin to adopt the Former Fat Girl way of eating— logging your meals, reading labels, pushing the bread basket away, and piling on the veggies—people are going to notice, and their reactions might be less than supportive. Secret #6 arms you with fixes to keep you true to your plan.

Chapter Six

Secret #6: Protect Yourself from
the Pushers

I was a major carnivore when I was a kid. Back in the 60s and 70s when I was growing up, the only people who went totally meatless were—gasp!—hippies. To our middle-class minds, abstaining from meat was a mark of deviance, evidence of a mind corrupted by marijuana and God knows what other controlled substances. At the very least it was just plain weird. No one in his right mind would refuse a platter of beef tips swimming in gravy or a juicy quarter-pound burger or a crispy fried chicken leg. In my world, dinner simply wasn't dinner without meat.

When I'd come home for the weekend during college, my dad would throw a couple of steaks on the grill as kind of a welcome home feast—a real treat when all you could afford on your student budget was ramen and boxes of mac and cheese. As the guest of honor, I'd get my pick of the platter. I always went straight for the cut with the thickest glob of fat along the edge. I'd carefully trim it off and pop the fat in my mouth. The rest of the family, who in my estimation didn't have palates sophisticated enough to appreciate the fine flavor of charred animal fat, would pass me their trimmings. Lucky me.

I tell you this not to disgust you (although I'm pretty sure I have) but to show you how completely alien I became to my family and friends when I stopped eating meat altogether a couple of years into my journey to Former Fat Girlhood. That was in the late 80s when the dangers of saturated fat had begun to ooze into the mainstream, and people began for the first time to realize that the fat that I so savored can plug up arteries like a hairball in a drainpipe. It was also around the time when weight loss gurus started counseling that counting fat grams was more important than counting calories. (Millions of pounds of Snackwell's cookies and one obesity crisis later, we know they were wrong.)

Anyway, in my own personal battle against dietary and bodily fat, I decided it was easier to banish meat altogether— beef, poultry, pork, everything but the leanest of fish—than try to downsize. Plus, when I really thought about it, I'd rather spend my precious allowance of calories on the carbs I so craved than on a hunk of sirloin. Well, you would have thought I'd had a sex change operation from the way my family reacted. They simply could not recognize this lap-running, dessert-shunning, pseudovegetarian as the daughter/sister/friend they had known all those years. They didn't know how to feed me anymore, and for my parents it almost meant they didn't know how to love me anymore.

Think about it: Those weren't just T-bones my dad was

serving during my weekend visits. They were love letters. Dad isn't anywhere near the stereotypical absent workaholic father, but he isn't the most emotionally communicative, either. He was using his Weber to show me how much he cared about me, how much he missed me, that I was still his little girl. And what did I do? I sent those thick, juicy, medium-rare expressions of his affection right back untouched. My meatlessness was the ultimate rejection.

I, of course, was oblivious to this stuff at the time. I was all wrapped up in working the Former Fat Girl program, trying to maintain the momentum I finally found through exercise, through INO, and all that. So I was completely unprepared for my parents' response to my whole new way of eating: They pushed. The first time I turned down the welcome home barbecue, they looked at me, stunned. It was like the air was sucked out of the room, like I'd uttered an ancient magical curse in some nonsensical Beelzebubian tongue. "Are you *sure*?" they asked. "What will you eat? Don't be silly. Just have a little." When I said no to spaghetti and meatballs, it was the same thing. When I didn't refuse a dish outright, they tried to heap a larger portion on my plate, almost desperately. They couldn't take no for an answer. Like a guy turned down by the woman of his dreams, my rejection only made them try harder. At every turn they tried to talk me into a slab of steak, to tempt me into going back on my word. It wasn't just meat, it was everything: our family's favorite cheesecake, the Entenmann's coffee cake I so loved, the creamy cheese dip we had on holidays.

It became a kind of tug-of-war: me on one side, struggling to pull myself out of my old Fat Girl life, and my family on the other, anchoring me to the place I was trying to escape. And it pissed me off.

Think about it: The decision to quit meat was far from

easy. I mean, I was the one who gobbled down not just the steak but the fat, too! It had taken me miles of running, millions of mantras, hours and hours of soul-searching to get strong enough to utter the word *no* and mean it. So you can imagine how I felt when I finally mustered up the will to pass up a slice of roast or a wedge of cake, only to have to deal with someone asking, "Are you *sure* you don't want any?" Not once but again and again and again. Every time they repeated the question, I could just feel my willpower weakening, just as a rope stretched beyond its limits begins to unravel and break, strand by strand, threatening to give way completely at any moment. "*Of course* I want some!" I wanted to yell. "But *it's not an option!*"

There were whispers that maybe I was developing some kind of eating disorder. The thought was ludicrous. Didn't they see that I already had one? I had been abusing food and abusing myself with food my whole life. My efforts to control the Fat Girl impulses that had essentially defined me were so out of character that the people around me didn't know what to think. But that was exactly the point. With my actions, with my running, with my "It's not an option," with my weighing and measuring, I was redefining who I was. What was out of character before was now in. And my parents, my siblings, and my friends just didn't get it. At least not yet.

They became Pushers—you know, like the guys who stand on street corners near the middle school offering contraband to innocent little kids lugging 50-pound backpacks and listening to God-knows-what on their MP3 players. My dad kept grilling the steaks, and my mom kept piling my plate with spaghetti and meatballs. And, at least at first, I was angry. Why didn't they want me to be happy?

* * *

This was not my first encounter with a pusher. My nana, my dad's mother, was a pro at it.

When I was in junior high, around seventh grade, I spent two weeks with Nana one summer that did a real number on my Fat Girl psyche. The family I babysat for, the one with the four kids, used to travel every summer to Washington, D.C., and Maine to visit relatives. The mom would fly up from Houston first with the kids (she didn't work, so she could take a longer break), the dad would meet them for a week or so, and then they'd all fly back together.

During one such trip, when the mom was pregnant with her fourth child and flying solo with three toddlers, their plane had to make an emergency landing, and she vowed never to fly again. So when the next summer rolled around, the family called and asked if I'd be up for a road trip. I'd keep the kids occupied in the car as the mom drove. We'd part ways in D.C. The dad would meet them later, as usual, and they'd all fly back together. Meanwhile, I would hop a train to visit my relatives in New York—Grandmom, my mom's mother, and my aunt Helen— and Nana in Philadelphia. Then I'd fly back to Texas alone.

It sounded like a great adventure. Helen was like a big sister to me, and she and her family lived close to the beach on Long Island. I had no doubt I'd have a blast there. And Grandmom lived in the city, so I'd get to hang out in Manhattan during my stay with her.

The only catch was that I'd have to give Nana equal time. At first glance you'd think Nana was the quintessential "fun grandma." In her cat-eye sunglasses she putted around town in a black '68 Camaro with a white racing stripe, not exactly what most sixty-something widows drove back in the mid-70s. She loved a good joke (even off-color ones, most of which she didn't completely get), and she was quite the party girl, always having luncheons and gatherings with a group of friends she referred to as "The Cousins," many of whom weren't related to her at all.

Nana might have been all fun and games with her friends, but around me she was a different person. She was hypercritical: From the clothes I wore to the foods I liked to the way I made my bed, Nana had an opinion on everything, and she didn't hesitate to share it. She wanted everything her way—no discussion, no dissension. Once when I was maybe four or five, I brought my favorite stuffed animal at the time—a two-foot-long floppy green snake—on a visit to Nana's beach house in Ocean City, New Jersey. Now, I can understand why a faux reptile might not seem to be an appropriate companion for a little girl, but Nana took her disapproval to the extreme. You'd think I was carrying around a shrunken head for all her nagging me to get rid of the thing—which, in fact, only made me cling tighter to it. So what did Nana do? She threw it out the window *in front of me.* She didn't hide it while I was on the beach, to see if I noticed it was gone (you know how fickle kids can be about toys); she didn't try to get me to trade for some more acceptable stuffed animal species. And, to make things worse, Nana's throwing arm wasn't good enough to clear the porch roof below, so there my poor snake landed, out of reach, to wither in the summer sun as I kept vigil.

You can see why I wasn't exactly crazy about staying with her for two weeks *alone*—no brother or sister or parent as a buffer. I felt like a delinquent being shipped off to military school. But there would be no road trip to D.C., no New York holiday, no I'm-so-grown-up plane trip alone if I wasn't willing to do the time at Nana's. So I packed my bags.

I'd like to say that it was better than I had imagined, but it wasn't. It was worse.

To be fair, Nana took me sightseeing, just like Grandmom and Helen did. Our itinerary was like something out of a Greyhound Bus tour brochure: We hit the Liberty Bell, Betsy Ross's house, Gettysburg—all the historical highlights. We ate stuffed crab and oozing, creamy Lobster Newberg at her favorite restaurants. We shopped at Wanamakers. We partied with selected cousins.

Why was I so miserable? The main problem—beyond the critical comments I knew were part of Nana's MO—was a little game she used to play, a game my dad refers to as Feed the Monkey and Watch Him Sh*t. Nana stocked her house with all kinds of junk food; she loved the stuff, candy especially. She would offer something to you—ice cream, doughnuts, cake, cookies, candy—push it on you, urge you to take more. And then, maybe a couple of hours or a day later, she'd say something like "Aren't those pants getting tight on you?" or "I think you've gained weight since you got here!" After that, she'd turn right around and ask you if you wanted a scoop of vanilla ice cream in your half cantaloupe—at *breakfast*—or a little more Coffee Rich (the nondairy half-and-half-like stuff that had as much fat in it as the real thing) on your cereal or a brick-size slab of crumb cake from the bakery down the street.

Once during my visit she took me to a 50s-type diner where the specialty was massive burgers and old-style ice cream fountain goodies, such as the gargantuan hot fudge sundae she urged me to order. As we were leaving, she said, "I probably shouldn't have let you have dessert, but I saw how your eyes lit up when the waiter walked by with one of those sundaes. I never *imagined* that you'd eat the whole thing!"

I burned with shame.

There were candy dishes all over the house: one for Hershey's Kisses, one for hard mints the color of blue topaz, one for M&Ms, and one for those caramels with the swirl of white sugary stuff in the middle. I don't have to tell you what happens when a kid encounters a candy dish: I took it as an invitation to indulge freely and frequently. After all, why would Nana put the stuff out if I wasn't supposed to eat it?

So I did. I started with the chocolate. I tried to nibble, not gobble—I did have *some* manners. When I had eaten about half of the M&Ms, I began working on the other candy. Maybe, I reasoned, my gluttony would be less noticeable if all the dishes were half full (the same logic I used to justify trimming away at a sheet cake, to even out the row). Of course she noticed. And of course she cared. And Nana wasn't the type to tiptoe around it, either. She was quick to point out the number of candy wrappers in the trash, the growing roll at my waistline, and my "astonishing" appetite for sweets.

But she kept refilling the candy dishes anyway. She kept buying the cookies and making the bakery runs. She kept pushing the junk on me, tempting me, testing me, and I failed every time. I resorted to sneaking the stuff upstairs to my room whenever I could, shoving it into my mouth when no one could see.

Even now, the self-assured Former Fat Girl that I am, it still hurts to remember how confused I was at the way Nana treated me. That summer vacation caused a rift in our relationship that lasted for years, and it only compounded the shame I already felt.

So you can see why I might have had some flashbacks when family and friends started with the pushing. Why, I wondered, would they want me to stay a Fat Girl forever?

Once I understood the whole "You are not like other people" thing, I got it. It wasn't that the Pushers wanted me to remain a Fat Girl because they didn't think of me as one in the first place. *I* was the one who wasn't content with the person everyone else saw from the outside—the way I looked, the way I acted. They just loved me for who I was.

Sure, they knew I was overweight, chubby, "husky" (awful term). It wasn't like they were blind. They teased me about it, even. But they had no idea what was going on inside. They didn't understand all the underlying emotions, all the secret shame I was carrying around, because unless you've been there yourself, you *can't* know.

They didn't get that I wasn't just trying to drop a few pounds or even a lot of pounds, I was trying to change my whole life. My family, Nana included, thought a piece of meat was a piece of meat; a hot fudge sundae was a hot fudge sundae. They didn't know that to me they were anchors, they were handcuffs, they were snares that were threatening to keep me from having the kind of life I wanted. They didn't know that my happiness, my vision of myself, my self-confidence were all tangled up in being a Fat Girl.

Figuring out that the Pushers didn't really intend to sabotage me made me less angry and frustrated, but it didn't change the reality I was dealing with: the temptation, the discouragement, and the doubt I sensed—all things that could derail my plan. Every time I pushed my plate away, the people I loved most felt as if I was pushing them away, just like I felt that they were pushing me back to that Fat Girl place when they tried to talk me into eating *just one meatball*. I had to figure out how to be the person I wanted to be, the person I was becoming, without threatening the people who loved the Fat Girl I was leaving behind.

*   *   *

Really, I had covered some of this territory before. I had kept my intentions a secret for as long as possible because I knew how other people can react when you start moving in an unfamiliar direction. I knew how scary that can be for them. But I couldn't hide it anymore. I was becoming a Former Fat Girl before their very eyes—physically *and* emotionally.

At this point my weight was steadily dropping. At the beginning of my stint on Weight Watchers, I was at about 150, and I dropped anywhere between 3 and 5 pounds a week. I actually started to look forward to my weekly weigh-ins. I couldn't wait to see how many pounds I'd lost. I couldn't care less about the meetings. I didn't need a cheerleading session; I got all the juice I needed from the scale, from the highs I got after I completed each run, from the way my clothes were fitting and my life in general was improving. Every week when I got the verdict from the Weight Watchers' official weigh-in person, it was like adding fuel to a fire. It stoked my motivation to stick to my daily "budget" of servings, to keep moving, to keep believing.

After the first four weeks or so, the weight loss slowed down; some weeks I lost half a pound, some weeks none. On weigh-in day I learned to wear the lightest clothes possible, no jackets, no lined wool pants, no big, embellished belts, no chunky earrings, no clunky shoes. I wanted to get credit for every ounce, to have a reason to give myself credit. Every weigh-in was an opportunity to celebrate, to pat myself on the back for a job well done.

I might sound superficial, vain, and overly focused on my appearance—and maybe I was, maybe I still am. But for me it was all connected. I wanted to feel good about myself, to feel more confident, to finally do something *just for me*—not to please other people but to please me. It had all started with running, which wasn't as much about getting to a certain weight as about the power surge I felt inside when I walked to my car, sweaty and satisfied, after each trip to the trail or the track. The scale had become another way to get that rush that comes when you see yourself getting closer to your goal.

My parents weren't the only ones who noticed the changes I was making and started pushing in response. Some of my closest friends gave me a hard time whenever I ordered my salad dressing on the side or the veggie burrito with no cheese or sour cream. It was almost as if my mere presence at the table made them defensive about what they were putting in their own mouths.

I first tried talking about it with them—explaining why, from the technical end, shunning slabs of animal fat (and flesh) was a good thing for me to do healthwise and weightwise. (Note the emphasis on me. I made it a point to avoid preaching or teaching. The last thing I wanted to do was become a Pusher myself.) I tried to explain that I couldn't eat a package of Pepperidge Farm Milano cookies for dinner or a bacon burger with cheese without beating up on myself, without feeling like a failure, without feeling perfectly humiliated. *It's fine for you*, I told them, *but I am not like you.*

Talking only went so far. My parents' restraint always seemed to wear off within a few days of our conversation, and they'd go back to pushing. I could see them biting their tongues as they gazed at what seemed to them like Barbie-doll-size portions of food on my plate. I could see them straining to keep from snatching up the serving spoon and forcing a glob of mashed potatoes on me. I could see the guilt in my friends' eyes as they picked at their desserts while I sipped a cup of decaf (with skim milk and Sweet 'n Low). Weren't we all raised to think that sharing is a good thing? And there I was, asking them not to.

When the going got tough—when I felt my resolve weakening under the pressure from the Pushers—I took the classic way out: I simply avoided them. I made some excuse not to eat with the friends who were most likely to make some crack about my dinner order. I cut back on my visits home.

The interesting thing was that I didn't have to resort to that too often. I had tools to help me stay focused on my goals, tools I had never had before. I had the power and self-confidence I'd built through exercise. I had INO. I finally knew in my heart that I was not like Becky, who could scarf down a box of cookies for dinner without feeling like a complete loser. I had seen a glimpse of the body I could have; I knew (approximately) how far I was from the finish line. For the first time in my life I was focusing on what *I* wanted, and I sure as hell wasn't going to let anything stand in my way. It was like I'd seen the purse of my dreams at a sample sale, and I was fighting tooth and nail to get to it before someone else snatched it up. I was willing to push, shove, and pinch my way through the crowd, through the distractions and temptations, through the cutting comments and criticisms that threatened to hold me back.

For once I was less concerned about disappointing everyone else than about disappointing myself. I was willing to risk what I had thought was the most precious thing—their love and approval—in the quest for my own happiness because I finally figured out that *my* happiness was what mattered most—not my parents', not my siblings', not my friends', and not my boss's. For too long I had placed more value on what the people around me thought and felt. Now it was my turn.

I had to choose between pleasing them—whoever "them" happened to be—and pleasing me.

I chose me.

So there I was, breaking out of my role as the self-sacrificing people pleaser and playing against type in pretty much every other area of my life, too. Take my job. I was working at the business weekly, struggling to hang on despite the abundance of grunt work I had to do (which included delivering bundles of issues to vendors around Austin out of the trunk of my beat-up Datsun). I had planned to finish my master's thesis on my off hours, but I couldn't muster up the motivation to even get started. As the months ticked away and my thesis went untouched, I realized that I was using it as a convenient excuse to stay in Austin and not go for that "real" magazine job I'd dreamed of.

I had to do something. In the same way I was cutting out the things in my life that had gotten my weight to an unhealthy high—the ice cream, the burgers, the fries—I had to cut myself loose from this anchor that was keeping me from taking that next career step. The thesis had loomed like a mountain in my mind; from a distance it looked formidable, forbidding, like you'd have to have superhero powers to scale it. That's how I used to see running five miles or losing 50 pounds. I could only imagine the before and after; I didn't have a clue about what to do in between, how to make it happen.

But I did now. I knew that five miles were twenty laps, and I could get there one lap at a time. I knew that losing 50 pounds was a matter of 2 pounds a week, and 2 pounds a week was a matter of six servings of bread a day or four servings of protein a day. You get the picture.

So I looked closer at that looming, scary mountain of a

thesis and began to make plans that would take me to the top. One was to reduce my hours at work. I figured I'd never get anything done if I continued to work from nine to five. So I proposed becoming a part-time investigative reporter at the business journal, keeping the stuff I liked about the job and leaving the grunt work to some unfortunate coworker. In my mind it was a win-win: My boss wanted us to stop kissing the local businessmen's butts and get more down-and-dirty stories in the paper anyway, and my plan would allow me to throw myself into the job. I boldly laid it all out for him, and he said no. He didn't like the part-time thing, didn't want to let me keep my benefits, yadda, yadda, yadda.

The funny thing was, I wasn't devastated, mortified, or humiliated. So he didn't go for it, so what? This was just a little bump in the road on the way to what I wanted. It was like one of those tough days on the running trail when I was hot or tired or both. What did I tell myself when that happened? It's not an option. It's not an option to quit because I just don't feel like running. It's not an option to let my boss's *no* stop me, either.

So I came up with Plan B. Needing some kind of steady gig to support myself, I talked to my old college professors about teaching a couple of classes a semester until I had the thesis done. The money stunk, I had no insurance, but I would try to do some freelance writing to fill in the gaps and piece together a life somehow. I held my nose, quit my safe, stable job with health and dental insurance and paid holidays, and jumped into the pool of financial insecurity with both feet.

And guess what? I didn't sink!

Oh, I was poor. Thank God for my Sears credit card; it fixed my car more times than I can remember. But I did it: I went out and hustled up pitifully paying freelance work. I entertained and instructed college students in the fine art of journalism as best I could. I pulled all-nighters in the University of Texas computer lab, inputting data, writing code, and pounding out results. Looking back from where I sit now, I see a different person from the Fat Girl I had been for so long. I was putting myself out there like never before—pitching stories to editors, creating lectures for my students, and tackling computer analysis as if it was second nature to me. At the time, though, I didn't think much of it, and that's a good thing. Because if I had stopped and thought too much, the old Fat Girl fears and insecurities would have come flooding back.

Put Your Happiness at the Top of the List

You probably know from all those previous attempts at losing weight that the most important people in your life aren't necessarily going to be your biggest cheerleaders, at least at first. You've heard the questions and the comments, the "That's *all* you're having?" And you hear every one of them as an expression of doubt, whether it's intended to be or not. It's so tempting to give in, to think "You're right. Why am I fooling myself? I can't change."

What's different is that this time you've already begun shoring up your self-confidence with exercise, with INO, and with all the Former Fat Girl fixes. You're not as fragile as you used to be. Taken together, the Former Fat Girl fixes create kind of a force field around you, so it's more difficult for the innocent comments (even sharply aimed arrows) to penetrate your heart, to prick your spirit, to wound your soul. That is, in a sense, what the Former Fat Girl plan is about: It's about building the mental and emotional toughness you need to succeed. It's about hacking into the Fat Girl programming that has determined your every move thus far and swapping in new Former Fat Girl code. (As you can see, I'm also fluent in computer geek.)

Still, you need specific tactics to deal with the Pushers because another thing that's different this time is your level of commitment—and the people around you can sense that. They can see you're serious about becoming a Former Fat Girl, and as you move in a new direction, they might begin to feel a little threatened. They start to realize that this time *you might just do it.* You might become that new person you've always wanted to become, and where would that leave them? They're afraid they won't recognize or relate to you anymore. And they love you just as you are; they don't understand why you have to change.

And then there are those in your life, family or friends, who might be Fat Girls themselves. They know what you're going through, but they might not be all that jazzed about your journey, either. They may see it as a reflection on them or even a betrayal. Your strength only makes their weakness more obvious. Your success only makes them feel more like failures.

While understanding all this can help you be more forgiving and less frustrated, you need concrete ways to stay strong when people and circumstances challenge you. I can help you steel yourself against the Pushers with My Former Fat Girl Fixes.

The Obstacle: How to Get the Pushers Comfortable with the Idea of the New, Former Fat Girl You

Sure, you care about the people around you, maybe too much. You can't expect yourself to simply flip a switch and turn off your compassion for them or your compulsion to please them. You need to find ways to reassure the people you love that you are not going to leave them behind—ways that don't involve your abandoning yourself and your Former Fat Girl plan altogether. Here's some advice that can help.

Former Fat Girl Fixes

No preaching.

Say your sister, your best girlfriend, your brother, or your husband could stand to learn a few lessons about portion control or exercise, or both. Fight the urge to climb aboard the Former Fat Girl soapbox. Even if you're careful to use a teaching tone, don't say a word unless you're asked. Preaching, teaching— whatever you want to call it—creates resentment among the Pushers, and resentment will only make them push harder. The no preaching fix even applies to those loved ones who are not Pushers but who are silently struggling with their own Fat Girl feelings. Remember how you reacted when someone foisted advice or information on you in the attempt to be helpful. Everyone has to come to it in his or her own time, in his or her own way, for his or her own reasons. A person may not be ready now and may never be, but the hope is that you do what you do quietly and inspire others and teach others without trying. What was it that Gandhi said? "Be the change you want to see."

Issue an invitation.

Consider this your best alternative to preaching. You need to let the people who love you know that you're not leaving them in your dust. So *don't*. Ask them to go with you. Maybe

your husband hasn't exercised since high school football practice twenty years ago, or the most strenuous thing your Mom
has ever done was cruise the sale racks at Bloomingdale's. Who
cares? Go ahead and ask them to walk with you or run with
you even if you think they'll turn you down. You'll get points
just for asking. The same goes for food: If they comment on
your veggie burger or grilled chicken breast, offer to fix one
for them. They might laugh or scoff, but so what? You've
made your point. You've let them know you still love them,
that you're not running (or walking) away. And, hey, you
never know: They might just take you up on it, and it might
just be fun.

Be careful who you brag to.

It's completely possible to be a braggart and not know it even
if you think you're the person least likely to blow your own
horn. I found that out the hard way. I had reached a new high
in my Former Fat Girl quest: I finally had a solid plan to get
where I wanted to be careerwise; my social life was hot; I had
a guy who might actually be interested in me as something
other than a buddy; and I had just bought a pair of size 5 jeans.
I was really and sincerely in awe of how things had turned
around, and, yes, I was proud of myself.

I was sharing all this one day with my friend Becky, my
closest girlfriend at the time. She and I talked about pretty
much everything, although now that I think about it, most of
it was complaining and kvetching. All of a sudden, while I was
describing my state of pure bliss, Becky let me have it. She said
that whatever guy I was talking about was *not* that into me, that
"anyone could be a writer," and how all I did was "rub her
face" in my happiness. I was stunned, utterly blindsided. Maybe
I could see how annoying it might be to hear me blather on

about how great my life was, but that wasn't really my style. And there was such venom in Becky's words. I was devastated at the idea that I couldn't celebrate my success and that she couldn't be happy for me.

Becky is a particular person and that was a particular situation, but that experience taught me a big lesson, one that will help you, too. You will have a lot to be proud of along your journey to Former Fat Girlhood. In your excitement, though, don't forget that some people might hear "I can't believe it! I lost 15 pounds!" as "You're a fat slob, and I'm not." That will only put them on the attack. Put yourself in their shoes (forgive the cliché). How would you feel if you were the one stuck in neutral while your friend, sister, or husband was zooming ahead in high gear? Hell, you might even know firsthand how it feels to be left behind. Never forget what it's like. Make it a point to stay mindful of where your friends and family members are in their own journeys so that you don't come off as insensitive. Remember, you were there once.

The Obstacle: Dating, Marriage, and Mommyhood: How to Deal with This Tricky Trio

Ah, if only we lived in solitary confinement; life would be so simple. No big, hulky men with big, hulky appetites; no kid-friendly snacks calling to you from the pantry; no crazy schedules besides your own to keep you from getting to the gym. What a life—a boring life—that would be. The men and kids in your life don't exactly have to be Pushers to make your journey to Former Fat Girlhood more complicated. Just the logistics of being in a household or committed relationship or seeking a committed relationship are challenges in themselves for wannabe Former Fat Girls. These tips will help you cope.

Former Fat Girl Fixes

Eat when you're with him.

It's true: Guys do like women who eat (just not too much). The fact that you enjoy food, within limits, says to him that you're open, sensuous, and adventurous. But that's not why you should eat with him. This is the time to do what you need to do for you, remember? Eat with him because food is a way of connecting, of celebrating. It's not the only way, but it's an important way. The dinner table is a place to get to know one another, to gather together as a couple or a family after a long day apart. So how do you stick to your plan when mealtimes can't be all about what you want (or need) to eat? If you're single and dating, use my "free day" fix. It saved me when I was going out with my now-husband Rick. I stuck to my healthy low-fat plan all week so I could let loose a little when we went out on Saturday night. I was also quick to suggest a restaurant. Rick has a fetish for barbecued ribs and cafeteria-style cooking, where the vegetables (if there are any) are either cooked in bacon grease, drenched in dressing, or swimming in butter. And wherever we went, I made it a point to order smart, ask a few strategic questions (Is there butter in the sauce? bacon on the salad?), and leave a few bites on my plate.

Now that we're married, I keep my diet under control by eating light during the day and saving my more substantial meal for dinner when our little family is all together. My breakfast might be oatmeal or cereal (occasionally a bagel as a treat); lunch is half a turkey or tuna sandwich, soup, or salad, maybe some baked chips, and fruit. Our dinners are healthy but more hearty: Pasta with shrimp, tomatoes, capers, and feta; pad Thai with lots of added veggies; grilled or barbecued chicken breasts (sans skin), potatoes (usually sweet for me), and salad; chicken tacos with fat-free refried beans, a sprinkling of low-fat cheese, and a dab of light sour cream and guacamole. Oh, and maybe a few tortilla chips on the side if I can dig out any folded ones from the bag. This ensures that Rick gets not just a satisfying meal but a healthy one, too, since he often indulges his meat tooth at lunchtime.

Suggest a moving date.

Who says you have to stick to the typical dinner and a movie? Dance. Hike. Rake leaves. Go bowling. Stroll through the botanical gardens—or the mall if he's the metrosexual type. Moving together can help you both relax and open up, so much so that some psychotherapists are hitting the walking trails with their clients instead of having them spend their sessions on the couch. You'll discover things about him that are hard to pick up in a dinner table conversation: how well you work together as a team, how he handles competition, what kind of work ethic he has, his inhibitions, and more. For married couples a moving date can keep the lines of communication open, something that's not always easy to do in the hectic day-to-day. See the sidebar on page 184 for more "moving date" suggestions.

Get him grilling.

Just about any guy can grill or at least thinks he can. Stroke his ego, call him the Grill Master, and he'll cook for you. You do the shopping: Buy him lean meats, light marinades, and even fish and veggies for a little challenge. Grilling is one of the healthiest, leanest cooking techniques; as long as you're not doing greasy burgers and hot dogs, you'll end up with a nice light entrée that he's just as happy to eat as you are. All you need to do is complement it with some healthy sides.

Practice patience post-pregnancy.

I didn't realize how much control I had before I had my son, Johnny—control over my time, my schedule, and the contents of my refrigerator. I'd say it was hard to adjust, but, really, the adjusting started when I was pregnant. As an "older" mom (I was thirty-nine when I got pregnant, forty when I delivered), I had to be careful, especially early on. I didn't exercise for the first trimester, afraid of having a miscarriage, and I was really too tired to do much anyway. I started running again at about three and a half months and was able to keep it up until about seven months when I thought I'd spare the trainers at the Y the anxiety of watching me on the treadmill, terrified that I would pop any minute.

I was fully prepared to spend the full nine months wrestling with my appetite and my willpower. Oh, I had my treats: McDonald's fries, the occasional dip cone from Dairy Queen, a Krispy Kreme doughnut hot from the oven. But I didn't go nuts on the junk. What I really wanted were fresh, cool foods such as salads, sushi (don't worry; I stuck with the cooked stuff), and avocado-tomato sandwiches on really grainy whole wheat bread.

Still, I gained forty-two pounds and had all that (and then some) to lose after Johnny was born in May 2001. But I wasn't in any shape to do anything about it for a good month or so. Without going into details, I had a fairly rough delivery. I needed time to heal physically, to get the rest I needed, to figure out just who this little being was and how to keep him happy. I wasn't like my friend Jill who went out bike riding

His-'n'-Her Workouts: Keep Him in Step with Your New Mind-set and Your Life

The greatest thing about being married or in a committed relationship (second only to never having to go on a blind date again) is having a man who loves you as you are. But for wannabe Former Fat Girls, a significant other can be more of a ball and chain than an agent for change. More than anyone your S.O. is likely to be afraid that when you lose the weight and get a life, you'll tell him to get lost. If he's not the active type, he may also become secretly intimidated by you the more comfortable you get in the weight room, at the track, or wherever. Asking him to exercise with you is a good idea, but you don't want to challenge him on his own turf. Here are some nonintimidating ways to ease him into exercising with you—to help him get used to the woman you are becoming, and realize that he will love the new you just as much as the old you.

Do it on your off days. If you're a Monday, Wednesday, Friday gal, ask him to take a stroll with you on one of your nonworkout days. You don't want to be worrying about how many calories you're burning (if he's not at your level). Your only goal should be to move together.

Keep it leisurely. Don't dress as though you're going for a workout. Throw your sneakers on with your jeans, for instance, instead of wearing Coolmax head to toe. If he's not the active type, this will reassure him that you're not out to kick his butt. If he's already a gym rat, dressing casually will keep him from running you into the ground and protect your fragile Future Former Fat Girl ego in the process.

Speaking of fun . . . No matter how good your skills at storytelling are, it's nearly impossible to make a fitness activity sound like fun to someone who just doesn't live in that world. (Trust me, I've tried.) So instead of trying to sell him on Spinning, which doesn't exactly sound pleasant when you try to describe it (pedaling to the throbbing bass of the Beastie Boys with a bunch of sweat-drenched strangers in a closet-size room filled with stationary bikes), invite him to do an activity that he already thinks of as fun. Bowling, for instance, or Ping-Pong, or even cycling (especially on a mountain bike; they're more kid-in-the-neighborhood than Tour de France). Show him that *exercise* doesn't always equal *pain* or *boring*.

And just in case you're curious, here's how many calories you can burn in an hour just by having fun!

Activity	For You Calories Per Hour	For Him Calories Per Hour
Air guitar	204	273
Bowling	204	273
Disco	374	500
Frisbee	204	273
Getting a massage	61	82
Giving a massage	272	364
Hot sex	102	136
Mini golf	204	273
Playing poker	102	136
Tag with the kids	272	384

with me two weeks after delivering her son. It took me a little more than a year to get my body back in Former Fat Girl fighting shape.

My best advice: Stay in touch with your body and give it what it needs, whether that's a ten-minute nap, a cracker and peanut butter to help keep the milk flowing, or a nice stroll in the sunshine. Treat yourself well by eating healthfully (it's better for the baby, too), and don't sacrifice sleep. And when you're ready, start moving again, taking it easy, using that 10 percent rule to propel yourself a little harder, a little further, but always taking a mental inventory of how you feel physically and mentally before you push on. Remember, it *can* be done.

Do what you can whenever you can.

I said it before: Just move. It doesn't have to be a workout, you don't even have to sweat. Getting your body in motion will burn calories, and when you're a superbusy mom, you have to take what you can get. For me that meant postpartum walks with Johnny in the Snuggly when I started feeling up to it. As he got older and I went back to work, our urban hikes became a weekend family ritual. We moved Johnny into a backpack, which I always insisted on carrying. I liked having him right at my ear where we could talk to each other, sing silly songs, and debate the names of bugs and trees. And the extra weight (we did this until he was about 30 pounds) helped me burn more calories. My husband, by the way, was happy to comply. This little strategy made activity a part of our family life early on, helping us build a nice little legacy that we've continued to carry forward.

Get the kids cooking.

Johnny has become my little sous chef (he even has his own little whisk). Enlisting his help when I'm making meals, even if it only involves sprinkling cheese on his chicken taco or stirring the cinnamon into his oatmeal, has gotten him excited about food, healthy food. He eats Thai, Chinese, and Mexican; he likes broccoli, carrots, squash, and salad. Sometimes I let him choose a special vegetable at the store, which he then can't wait to cook and taste. What's this have to do with *your* diet? Well, getting your kids excited about healthy food means you'll have more of it around.

Buy snack packs.

Kids are born snackers. If you put a box of Teddy Grahams in front of them (especially the chocolate ones), they'll be gone before the SpongeBob theme song is over. I'll bet you, though, that if you gave them a lunch box snack pack, they'd gobble it down and be satisfied for a lot fewer calories (only 150 per bag). And if they're not, you can steer them to a snack from the other food groups—an apple, a tube of yogurt, a low-fat string cheese. All these mini versions of tasty treats don't just make it easier to pack their lunches in the morning, they're automatic portion control for you. Somehow it's much harder psychologically to break open another bag of mini Oreos when you've just polished one off.

The Obstacle: The Pain You Feel at the Pusher's Lack of Support

One thing that's not part of the Fat Girl programming is a spam filter—one of those things that keep stuff like ads for sexual enhancements and mortgage loans from cheesy companies from piling up in your e-mail in-box. It's as if you need one of those to help you filter out the junk that can distract you from your goal, that can undo all the work you've done. You are programmed to take completely to heart every expression of doubt (or what you perceive to be doubt) and every hint that the people around you aren't on board with your quest for Former Fat Girlhood. Even innocent remarks can be wounding, devastating. That's true no matter the source, but especially when your inner circle is sending the messages. How to deal? Read on.

Former Fat Girl Fixes

Lower your expectations.

What made it so hard for me when I started getting pushback, especially from my parents, was that I expected them to be supportive right out of the gate. I didn't see it coming: the "Now, Lisa, you just aren't eating enough. You're going to make yourself sick!" and the "What's with all this running? You'd better watch it, or you'll end up with arthritis!" But later on it all made sense (like everything usually does from a distance). They were not afraid that I would catch a cold or sprain my ankle or even become anorexic; they were afraid that the Lisa they knew was disappearing. And they didn't know who would come along to replace her. Doesn't that sound familiar? That's kind of like the fear that kept me from changing all those years.

Remove the element of surprise, and you'll have it a lot easier than I did. *Expect* your loved ones to push. *Expect* them to act as if they don't want you to do the exact thing you thought they wanted you to do for years—lose the weight, that is. *Expect* them to seem to want to sabotage you (and know that they don't mean it). If you have your guard up from the beginning, you're less likely to be knocked cold by a sucker punch.

Remember: It's all about them.

When someone else wronged me for whatever reason, I used to think "*I* would never do that! *I* would never act like that! *I* would never treat someone like that!" And then I discovered over time that people do many things that hurt others without intending to. That's probably not news to you, but it's worth reminding yourself that the Pushers are probably acting out of self-interest, that what-about-me place, and not really conspiring to keep you from getting the life you want. I still struggle to keep this on top of my mind to help me undercut my tendency toward this kind of knee-jerk self-righteousness.

Practice selective hearing.

If you have a child over the age of three or a husband, you no doubt have seen selective hearing at work. Men and children have a particular knack for hearing only what they want to hear. (That's just one among a long list of similarities between the two.) Even when you are standing nose to nose, making eye contact, and the Spiderman video or ESPN chatter is turned off, they have a way of missing the most important nuggets of a conversation. Learn from them. I believe in girl power and all that, but there are a lot of things we can steal from the men in our lives—like how not to think about things too much (or at all), how to ask for what we want without having to have a life coach prompting us from the sidelines, and how to feel like a rock star naked, even though you may look more like bloated old Elvis.

When in doubt, laugh.

Don't get me wrong: I know how hard it is to keep your head up when it feels like everyone's working against you. I know how hard it is not to react, not to take it personally, to let comments slide off you like an omelet (egg whites only, please) from a nonstick pan. I know because I had (and continue to have) a particular issue with this. An ex-boss and great friend, Pam, used to tell me that I needed to learn how to "control my face." If I was angry, hurt, annoyed, confused, or whatever, you could see it by the flash in my eyes, the particular furrow in my brow, the shape of my mouth. After about seventeen years of practice, I've gotten better, but it's still a struggle. One of the things I've learned along the way is that it's better to laugh off a comment than to defend yourself with some kind of clever quip. *Clever* often comes off as defensive, and you really don't want to get into a name-calling match now, do you? Giving a little chuckle with some vacant look in your eyes is always better.

I use this tactic even now as a Former Fat Girl because the funny thing about finally getting where you want to be weight-wise is that people actually comment on what you eat more openly than they do when you're overweight. To wit: One day I was at the office, hitting the break room refrigerator for my 3:00 P.M. snack of baby carrots. A woman I worked with, Cindy, was pulling something off the printer in the same room (we were a little cramped for space). Cindy was a big woman— very tall, I would say five feet ten, and had some weight issues of her own. When she saw my little bag of carrots, she said in a light but sarcastic tone, "Ooooh, Lisa! Doesn't that look yummy? Now, don't indulge *too* much." I let out the little chuckle that I reserved for such an occasion. But I was thinking, *What makes it okay for people to criticize what I'm eating?* If she was digging into a bagful of Double Stuf Oreos, would I have said, "Ho, Cindy, hitting the cookies a little hard today, are we?" No. I wasn't even tempted to deliver such a stinging comeback due to my own Fat Girl history. But I might have tried to defend myself or explain myself, which would probably have turned into a conversation I didn't want to have (see No Preaching, above). The chuckle response saved me from all that. It will save you, too.

Keep your eyes on the prize.

Okay, so you have all the tools from chapter 4 to help you see the Former Fat Girl you will soon (!) be. *Do not forget them.* This is not a linear process. All the Former Fat Girl secrets work together to get you where you need to be—and keep you there. That's one thing. Another is to come up with a visualization to protect yourself from all the distractions, traps, and potholes that can trip you up on your way to your goal. Mine was straight from (don't laugh) the Bible. You know the story about Peter walking on the water? He had seen Jesus taking a stroll out there in the waves, and in a what-the-heck moment he went out to join him. He was getting the hang of it when all of a sudden he looked around and it dawned on him: *Wait, this is nuts! I can't be doing this! I'm breaking the law of physics!* Then he began to sink. Once Peter looked back into Jesus' eyes, he started rising back to the surface so he could complete his own little miracle.

Now, non-Christians, please forgive my digression. My point is not to proselytize. My point is to show you how I used visualization to keep me focused. I'm Peter, taking my shaky steps toward the vision I have of myself as a Former Fat Girl (aka Jesus). As soon as I drop my gaze, the enormity of what I'm doing gets to me: the swirling doubts and fears of myself and others, and the magnetic pull of the kitchen and the couch. That's when I start to sink. I could *feel* it happening. And I could feel myself rising up, standing straighter, and feeling stronger when I envisioned Jesus' eyes willing me forward, drawing me to my future as a Former Fat Girl.

That parable is so powerful for me that I still use it whenever self-doubt or seemingly impossible circumstances threaten to drag me down. It might not work for you, but you can create your own story or find one that speaks to your own spirit.

Choose you. Choose you. Choose you.

Do I need to say anything else? This is *your* time, *your* program, *your* future. You have to stop sacrificing your happiness for the sake of others. If you need my permission, you've got it. Put "Choose you" Post-its on your refrigerator, on your computer monitor, on your dashboard, on your workout bag. Repeat it like a mantra so you won't forget it when you're faced with a decision that might disappoint someone you love. And don't forget: *You* are someone you love, too. Don't you deserve the same consideration you so willingly give to everyone else?

Choosing you doesn't mean you're selfish. It doesn't mean you love the people in your life any less. It's putting yourself in the right place on your list of priorities: at the top. As much as Secret #6 is about protecting yourself from the push and pull of other people, it's also about knowing what you want and standing your ground. Knowing, for instance, that you want to squeeze in an early-morning workout twice a week and leave your husband in charge of the kids—and not letting the fear that he might be put out or pissed off keep you from even asking. It's knowing that you don't have to go for seconds of your mom's meat loaf *just to be nice*. It's knowing in your heart that one serving is enough, that you don't need more, and trusting that knowledge enough to say no, no matter how many times you're asked. Otherwise, you're drifting in the air like a half-dead helium balloon, ready to sail across the room at the slightest tap.

The next and last secret, lucky #7, gives you the key to cultivating the attitude you need to earn yourself permanent status as a Former Fat Girl. It's this attitude that will help you bounce back from the kinds of setbacks in your life, emotional or otherwise, that might have sabotaged your weight loss attempts in the past or caused you to gain in the first place. Intrigued? Read on.

Chapter Seven

Secret #7: Happiness Lives
in the Uncomfort Zone

I'm no genius, but I did display a gift for math at a very early age. By the time I was four, I'd already mastered my first algebra equation: Food + Infinity = Fun. My idea of a good time always involved eating, and the more (on my plate, that is) the merrier.

Eating out was always a special treat because we didn't do it all that often. For one thing, it simply wasn't practical for my parents to take the five of us kids out much on my dad's salesman salary. When we did venture out for the rare restaurant experience, I was determined to get as much out of it as possible. To me that meant eating until I was practically doubled over in pain. If my stomach wasn't aching by the time the check came, the evening was a waste.

I remember eating at a seafood restaurant with the family when we lived outside Boston. Huge platters of fried every-thing (shrimp, fish, clams, oysters, you name it) served with—you guessed it—french fries. I stuck to the shrimp and maybe a stuffed crab (shells filled with a buttery breadlike concoction, only a trace of crabmeat in it), dutifully cleaning my plate, stomach cramping under the load. Ignoring the pain, like a football player who scrambles for the goal line despite the bone-crushing blows from the defense, I'd snatch up the des-sert menu to place my order and practically scrape the design off the plate to make sure I got every last bit.

That was typical of the way I behaved in restaurants—not to mention at major holiday meals and other special occasions involving food—until my quest for Former Fat Girlhood. When I was invited to parties, I cared less about who was on the guest list than what was on the menu. I judged the success of every occasion by the food: weddings (all about the buffet), birthdays (the cake—icing in particular—was the star attrac-tion), holidays (Christmas, cookies; Easter, candy; Halloween, the size of the haul). And in my everyday life I used food to make bad (or even mediocre) days better.

So you can see why I reacted to the idea of going on a diet with complete and utter dread. I wasn't one of those girls for whom a lo-cal regimen is simply inconvenient and annoying, who see the needle on the scale moving in the wrong direction and think, "Well, damn. I guess it's salad for me tonight." To me it was much, much more. A diet robbed me of my favorite way to pass the time, the primary source of joy in my life, the only way I had back then to relate to and connect with other people. Just thinking about it made me want to quit before I even started—which I did many, many times.

Think about it this way: Putting me on a diet was like telling someone who loved to paint that she could never pick up a brush again or—even worse—that from now on she could use only the color brown. No yellows, reds, blues, or purples— nothing but dull, drab brown.

Some painters would say forget it. How can you be an artist without color? Why even try? But another might say, after wrestling her way through the five stages of grief, "Well, let's see what I can do with brown." She might take the limits placed on her, the new restrictions on her life, as a challenge, not a defeat. She might discover and experiment with the many variations of the color, from light pine to mahogany. And she might end up with a canvas she is proud of and satisfied with— maybe even one she loves better than anything else she's ever done—as much because of the end result as what she had to go through to get there.

That, ladies, is exactly what happened on my journey to becoming a Former Fat Girl. I had to repaint my life with a whole new color palette; I had to live within a new set of rules. As I've told you, it was hard to do at first. I fought. I whined. But I could see it. Deep down I knew that I was fooling myself. Food *wasn't* fun. Food *wasn't* nurturing or comforting. It *wasn't* self-love. It *wasn't* other-love—not the way I used it. It was keeping me stuck in my "big-boned" body, in my second-rate jobs, in my always-the-friend-never-the-girlfriend love life. It was keeping me stuck in that comfortable place that I so wanted to escape.

I knew what I had to do. I had to make myself *un*comfortable. Every time I took a risk—walking into that Jazzercise class, lacing up my running sneakers, saying no to a slab of steak (and yes to me and what I wanted), quitting my job to finish my thesis—I felt one step closer to true happiness. It's as if I had an internal dimmer switch: With every victory over fear, every move out of that cushy comfort zone, the light got a little bit brighter—and the scarier the thing, the brighter the light grew.

I became like that painter who embraced her new, earthy palette. I started looking at this whole new life as an adventure, not a prison sentence. I started to believe I could find new ways to have fun, to find comfort, to feel satisfied, to be truly happy—ways that didn't involve stuffing myself. And I set out to explore.

My first frontier was the kitchen. My mission: to find healthy, diet-conscious food that didn't taste like punishment on a plate. I started devouring "light" cookbooks, poring through recipes, trying dish after dish. I made my share of duds, mind you; most of the time they were the result of misguided recipe tinkering on my part. I learned the hard way not to try to strip all the fat out of a dish, ending up with casseroles that were watery instead of creamy; scones you could use for door stoppers; and crustless, yolkless quiches that disintegrated into a soupy mess when you tried to cut them. If you've ever tried to make bran muffins without any oil, you know what I'm talking about. The outcome was less like a breakfast food and more like concrete.

But I also found a good many winners. For instance, I discovered that lasagna tastes just as decadent made with low-fat ground turkey, light cottage cheese instead of ricotta, and about half the gooey mozzarella that is in most standard recipes. I'd make a batch every couple of weeks, carefully cutting it into the proper-sized portions (as dictated by WW) for freezing. I looked forward to my lasagna nights as much as I used to look forward to Mom's spaghetti and meatballs.

As I searched for new, lighter takes on my old food friends,

I discovered tricks I could use to slim down favorite family recipes, like my Nana's yummy cheesecake, which is just as yummy made with low-fat cream cheese and sour cream, and two egg yolks instead of three. At the same time I tried to make these dishes work a little harder in the nutrition category by adding or subbing in healthier ingredients. I tried whole wheat flour in Mom's applesauce bread with decent results and started using whole wheat pasta, bread, and tortillas whenever I could. I stuck to safe territory, playing around with recipes I knew I liked rather than trying to talk myself into adding weird stuff like tofu to my repertoire. I didn't want to shock my system too much; after all, a large pepperoni with extra cheese was only a phone call away.

I took on this culinary challenge as if I were in some Betty Crocker calorie-conscious cook-off. I actually started to have fun. Cooking was not just an excuse to lurk in the kitchen, hoping for a stray crumb or dollop of cookie dough. It was like a game with a new set of rules and a new way to win. Winning wasn't just about pleasure, and it wasn't at all about quantity. To win I had to create food that I would truly enjoy, that would leave me satisfied, within the Former Fat Girl framework.

I began eating foods as "naked" as possible—with as little salt, fat, sugar, or creamy sauces as they needed. I experienced flavors in their truest senses—the buttery effect of certain lettuces, dressed with a drizzle of oil and vinegar instead of a flood; the candylike sweetness of homegrown tomatoes unmasked by salt; the brightness of a Ruby Red grapefruit, no sugar necessary.

Along the way something physical started to happen. I began to *prefer* my Former Fat Girl food to the stuff I used to eat. I became so used to my new way of eating that I could tell when a particular dish went too far in the sweet, fat, and/or salty direction. And not only that, I didn't like it. It became easier and easier for me to say no to Mom's green bean casserole with incredibly salty cream of mushroom soup or a scoop of mashed potatoes whipped with liberal amounts of butter and cream. I don't have to tell you what a breakthrough that was. Without knowing what I was doing, I had reprogrammed my palate. I was now the proud owner of a set of Former Fat Girl taste buds—and it felt great.

At the same time I was inching out of my comfort zone fitnesswise, too. In this new world of mine, skipping exercise was INO, remember? Exercise can get boring if you stick with the same-old same-old, so I started mixing things up, but not too much. I had finally established a real fitness routine, and I didn't want to do something stupid and turn back into the couch potato I used to be.

By this time I had worked up to running five miles several days a week on that dusty quarter-mile track where I'd first laced up my jogging shoes. Five miles—twenty laps—had been my goal. If I could make it that far, I thought, I might be able to handle the jogging trail around Town Lake where all the "real" runners in Austin put in their miles. I was nervous about going from the track to the trail, though, and not just because I might not fit the profile of a "real" runner. I loved the way my track runs were neatly split into manageable chunks; each lap was short enough that it made the entire thing seem doable and was occasion for a mini-mental celebration. (Yea! Three down, two to go!) In comparison, the trail was one loooong-ass lap. Would it be interminable? Would it be unbearable? Would I give in to the whiner in my head and go back to my old Fat Girl ways?

Physically, I was ready. Mentally? I wasn't so sure. But I decided to try anyway. I told myself that this first time was a reconnaissance mission—not an official workout, just a jaunt around the lake. I tried to keep my expectations low; the last thing I wanted was to end up feeling like a loser.

As I loped along, I discovered a small bridge that crossed over a feeder to the lake about a half mile in. Then, after another half mile, there was a second bridge. Then another mile or so away, a third. I think there were five bridges total along the route. I had found my new landmarks, my new signposts on the way to the finish line. Instead of "three laps to halfway, two laps to halfway," my mental litany became "three bridges to halfway, two bridges to halfway." That and my strategic purchase of an FM Walkman radio stifled the whiner and made me a regular at the Town Lake trail.

My budding reputation as a jock may have boosted my ego and marked a massive shift in my self-image, but it didn't do much for my love life. Don't get me wrong, I had become popular with the guys. In fact, during that time of my life, I probably had more male friends than female friends. But my behavior on the court and on the field just fueled the backslapping, punch-in-the-arm way I related to the men in my life.

It's not as if I hadn't made any progress, though. I finally had my first sexual experience at the ripe old age of twenty-six, a supremely awkward, extremely unemotional encounter that I suspect was prearranged by my friend Gabriele (although I never asked; I really don't want to know). If I merely mentioned a guy, Gaby would ask, "Did you f*** him?" I think she thought that having sex would forever change my life, which it didn't, but, hey, it was worth a try. If there was anything I was *un*comfortable about, it was sex. That's the attitude with which I fell into bed with Sean.

Sean was probably—no, definitely—the most promiscuous man I had ever met (I have since known others who would rival him). He came off as kind of a jerk, but I had a soft spot for jerks, and I think he truly did love women. We had been around each other in group situations, but I don't think we even talked that much until he called to ask me out. Even so, it didn't surprise me. It was as if I knew that there was some back-room deal for him to deflower me that night. Maybe I was just having a flashback to high school, to my innocent fling with George because it was my turn, or to my senior prom suitor, a guy who had pulled my name off the Still Dateless list as the magic night loomed. It wasn't that Sean had chosen me for who I was; I was next in line.

I don't even remember much about the whole thing. We must have first gone to see a movie or something. I don't think we went out to eat (I would definitely have remembered that).

However it happened, we ended up at his house, in his bed. Since Sean didn't drink, I abstained, too, so I didn't even have a nice dreamy buzz to take the edge off. There was a complete and utter lack of chemistry between us, which didn't help at all with the mechanical side of things, if you know what I mean. There was some requisite kissing, I think, and I remember stripping down to bra and panties with the lights off, scrambling under the sheets so he couldn't actually see what he was getting into.

It was obvious he had done this kind of thing before—not just the sex part but the sex-with-a-Fat-Girl-virgin part, too. There wasn't much talking between us, and when it was over, he stayed in bed just long enough. And then he left the room so I could dress and rearrange myself without a spectator.

I wasn't particularly traumatized by losing my virginity with someone I barely knew, someone I was certainly not in love with. I didn't even feel guilty, despite all that good-girl Catholic breeding. I remember taking my mental temperature to see if I felt any differently now that the act was over. Was I more girly, more flirty, less sisterly? Hardly.

No, that single sexual act didn't lift the spell I was under—the You're a Fat Girl, Who Could Love You? spell. But as I continued to lose the weight and work my Former Fat Girl program, I found myself straying out of the safety zone I had created around me that insulated the woman inside from any kind of serious relationship with a man.

I did sleep with Sean a second time in case I missed something on the first go-round. But, no, there was no life-changing moment. I did go on other, equally awkward dates and blind dates, none of which culminated in nights of sexual passion (or any kind of sex, save a handful of somewhat enthusiastic make-out sessions with a guy whose name I can't even remember). But as lackluster as my love life was, at least I did finally have something resembling one. Just the fact that a guy would ask me out was a sign, I thought, that maybe I was a little more open to the whole experience. For one thing, I started recognizing those little hints guys drop, those comments they cast into the air hoping to get a nibble, such as "Hey, do you like sushi?" and "Have you heard about that new Stallone movie?" Now I recognized them for what they were—date bait—whereas before I was completely oblivious.

And then I met a man I could actually see myself married to, and not in that Davy Jones daydreamy way. David was perfect on paper: smart, funny, kind of creative (he played the guitar), fairly open-minded, and kind of a jerk but kind of sensitive at the same time. And there definitely was a spark between us, the same kind of spark I'd had with John, the boyfriend of a best friend in high school on whom I secretly had a crush.

We could talk about important things: politics, music, art. I made him laugh, and he made me laugh. But here's the difference: John was taken; David was not. David was a real possibility, not someone safe with a risk-free guarantee.

But something happened—or should I say *didn't* happen—between us. We did all the things couples do: We went out, the two of us, alone. We rode bikes together. We picked out and decorated his Christmas tree. We went to concerts and clubs. I met his parents and his sister. But we never got physical; we never even kissed, not once. That stupid cliché about "ships passing in the night," that was us. There was a moment that came and went, a missed opportunity without my knowing. And I couldn't get it back, no matter how hard I tried and how long I held on. We remained friends, but friends were all we were ever going to be. It took me years to figure that out. I know I wasn't completely free of my Fat Girl programming, or I would at least have asked him why. I would have pushed the issue—like I did when I met my husband years later. I slipped my business card to him when I was on a blind date with someone else (but that's another story).

I was at an uncomfortable place in my career, too. Finally finished with my master's thesis after two extensions on the standard six-year deadline, I was free of the anchor that had kept me in Austin. I had no excuse for staying anymore.

I wasn't ready to leave, though—not just yet. This time it wasn't because I was afraid to go. Caught up in my newfound spirit of adventure, I had gotten it into my head that I didn't really want a job at a magazine. I didn't want to be bound to one particular desk in one particular office at one particular place. What I really wanted was to move to New York City and be a freelance writer, to flit from assignment to assignment, writing about whatever I was interested in at the time. I would travel the country—maybe even the world!—notepad in hand, getting the story, whereever and whatever it was.

What was I smoking? I mean, freelancing was the complete opposite of those safe, secure, albeit boring jobs I had taken so far. No insurance, no Friday payday, no 401(k). The only job riskier would be as an image consultant for Courtney Love.

I look back fondly at my naïveté. To actually think I could snag plum assignments at *Vogue* or *Harper's* with my meager publishing credentials? But as crazy as it sounds now, this pipe dream of mine represented a major turnaround. Until then my Fat Girl programming would have kept me from even considering such a thing. I finally believed in myself enough to not only daydream about the life I could have but actually get off my butt and do something about it.

I may have been ignorant, but I wasn't stupid. I knew it would take money—a good deal of money—to make that kind of move. I wasn't going to get to New York on what I made as a part-time teacher and a twenty-five-cents-a-word freelancer in Austin. So I set about getting a job, any job, as long as the pay was good. I planned to save every penny I could, head northeast, and proceed to knock on the door of every editor in Manhattan.

I took a job in the public information office at the state welfare department in Texas, a job I knew was way too easy for me almost immediately, just like all the other jobs I'd had. But this time was different. This time I wasn't choosing out of fear or weakness. This was a calculated choice; this was part of the plan. This time the job wasn't just another dead end; it was a beginning.

I plugged away as a state employee for about a year and a half, working on ad campaigns to recruit foster parents and writing stories for the employee magazine (one of which was killed because I had described the lives of the welfare clients "too vividly," which I took as a compliment). I struggled to write pamphlets on preventing sexually transmitted diseases for women who could barely read. It was more of a challenge than I thought it would be.

But I wouldn't let myself settle. I had a plan. In addition to scrimping and saving and fantasizing about some third-floor walk-up three-way studio share in Manhattan, I cruised the job boards in the journalism school placement office every chance I got, and scoured the help-wanted ads in the national trade rags (this is what we did before we had Monster.com). Even though I dreamed of the freelance life, it wouldn't hurt to see what kind of staff jobs were out there, right? After toying briefly with the idea of applying for an opening at the *National Enquirer* (What the heck? The pay was great, and I could write about aliens!), I saw the perfect thing: a posting for a senior editor at the largest health and fitness magazine in the country.

Okay, so, forget that I had no background in health, only that I didn't get sick all that often, and when I did, I went to the doctor. Forget that the only stuff I knew about fitness was what I learned trying to get myself up and moving. Forget that, ahem, I'd never even *seen* the largest health and fitness magazine in the country. I slapped together a resume and a somewhat irreverent cover letter. (It started with a little poem: You want healthy, you want fit, you want creative . . . I think I'm it!) When I slid the oversized envelope into the slot at the post office, I remember actually thinking, *Okay, here we go! This could change my whole life!*

I didn't think about it too much—about my chances, about freelancing and all that. I didn't have anything to lose except maybe that surge of self-respect that washes over you every time you reach for what you think is impossible.

Four or so years before—before I discovered Jazzercise and made "It's not an option" my mantra and all that—I would never have ripped out that ad. For one thing, I didn't exactly look the part. But not only that, I wouldn't have had the courage to even think I could try.

I was scared to death. It did flash through my head when I still had a grip on the envelope that I could waste the postage, throw the thing out, and forget the job. After all, who was I to think I could be an editor at a national magazine? But then again, who was I to think I could be a runner? Who was I to think I could stop at one bite of chocolate cake? Who was I to think I could wear low-rise jeans, show some leg, dance by myself?

All those things were scary, but I let go of that fat manila envelope, of the scary "what ifs." I couldn't allow that ad to go unanswered. I knew the things that made me the most afraid, the most uncomfortable, were the things that would make me the happiest. I *had* to do it. I had been comfortable for too long.

Find the Uncomfort Zone

You might notice that I haven't bored you with a pound-by-pound recount of how much weight I lost during my journey to Former Fat Girlhood. That's not some kind of editorial oversight; it's intentional. Because being a Former Fat Girl isn't about what size you wear or how many pounds you lose. It's more about how you think about yourself; how you go for what you want; how you take risks and speak up; how you walk through life with your chin up; how you look people in the eye when you speak.

Now, I'm proud of the fact that I no longer have to bypass the cool clothes on my way to the "big girl" section of the department store. I'm happy (and, frankly, still amazed) that I can order crème brûlée without feeling that everyone in the restaurant is pitying me. I know what a victory it is to be sitting here, a bona fide Former Fat Girl in body *and* mind. My point is, though, that reshaping your body isn't what makes you a Former Fat Girl. Even if you lose the weight by dieting and exercise, until you work on your head, until you work through that Fat Girl programming, there's a good chance you'll go back to your old ways. You know what I'm talking about— that yo-yo exercise so many of us have been through. All those times when you tried to "be good," when you adopted the diet or fitness flavor of the week. Sure, you might have lost weight and might even have reached your "goal," but unless you also shed that Fat Girl persona along with the pounds, that needle on the scale will start creeping back up again.

To truly become a Former Fat Girl, your goal can't be merely a number on a scale or a size on a clothing rack because this isn't just a diet: You are creating or *re*creating the life you want to live. In a way it's like moving into a new neighborhood or a new city. You've got to find a new route to work, a new grocery store that carries all your favorite stuff, a coffee shop where the house blend is just strong enough and the vibe isn't too annoyingly hip. You can't do things the old way— that's the rule. There's no use bitching about it, so you might as well suck it up, get out there, and explore. In trying to become a Former Fat Girl, you're living in a town where not exercising is INO, where fun and food aren't synonymous, where there's no Fat Girl façade to hide behind. Sometimes it might feel more like you've been banished to a foreign country

Six Hot Spas for Former Fat Girls

Where can you go to jump-start your Former Fat Girl journey? Try these destinations. Each of these spas offers a cocktail of fun fitness activities, great calorie-conscious food, and valuable advice and inspiration to get you going. And their easygoing atmospheres make everyone feel welcome.

1. **Green Mountain at Fox Run, Ludlow, Vermont.** This mountain retreat for women only focuses on weight loss in a gentle, realistic way. Its non-diet program focuses on fitness, sensible eating, and a healthy body image. (Details at www.fitwoman.com.)

2. **Red Mountain Spa, St. George, Utah.** A two-hour drive from Las Vegas, Red Mountain is the prime spot to explore all your fitness options. Who wouldn't get jazzed about hiking, mountain biking, or just moving in the canyons of South Utah? (Details at www.redmountainspa.com.)

3. **Lake Austin Spa Resort, Austin, Texas.** Great (light) food, complete with cooking classes, a fabulous variety of fitness activities, and the ultimate pampering under the Texas sun. Lake Austin has expanded in recent years, but its laid-back, slightly rugged Hill Country undertones endure. (Details at www.lakeaustin.com.)

4. **Rancho La Puerta, Tecate, Mexico.** Eat food fresh from the on-site organic farm, hike the meadows and mountains, and literally get away from it all (no TV, no phones) at this mind-body hideaway just an hour from San Diego. (Details at www.rancholapuerta.com.)

5. **Canyon Ranch, Tucson, Arizona, and Lenox, Massachusetts.** The mother of all spas, Canyon Ranch might conjure images of uptight, skinny, metabolic mutants, but there are plenty of us normal girls among the clientele. The cuisine is top-notch (and there are classes so you can learn to make it at home), the fitness offerings are cutting edge, and the on-site professionals can offer you quality advice. Sign up for the Optimal Weight Management program for specific advice and attention. (Details at www.canyonranch.com.)

6. **New Age Health Spa, Neversink, New York.** One of the country's more affordable options for spa goers, New Age Health Spa is set on 280 rambling acres in the Catskill Mountains, a quick jaunt from New York City. From the fully equipped gym to the Pilates and yoga classes and to year-round outdoor activities (hiking in the summer, snowshoeing in the winter), it's easy to get moving here. Indulge in the signature Maple Sugar Body Polish (remember, it's New England) and meals made with *über*healthy produce grown in the spa's own greenhouses. (Details at www.newagehealthspa.com.)

where you don't speak the language—it sure did to me—but the Former Fat Girl tools will give you the strength to keep going.

It will feel a little strange. It *should* feel a little strange. After all, you're breaking new ground, you're busting out of your rut, you're taking that comfort zone you've been hiding in for so long and tearing it wide open. You're experiencing the thrill of the Uncomfort Zone.

Comfort used to be what you looked for, but now it's your enemy. You will start seeing challenges all around you, little things like speaking up at a meeting, initiating a conversation at a party or on a plane, or confronting an issue face-to-face rather than via e-mail. Situations you would have been oblivious to before will become hurdles you are driven to jump. And the funny thing is, if you don't jump them—if you break step and go around—you'll feel weird. You'll feel like you wimped out. And wimping out was normal—until now.

When that happens—when you wimp out and a little voice inside your head calls you on it—that's when you know you're truly living the Former Fat Girl way. You'll hear it when you stifle the question you're dying to ask. You'll hear it when you say, "That's okay," when it's really not. You'll hear it, too, when you skip your workout for no good reason or eat something you don't even like all that much just because it's there. That's how the pounds will come off.

From where you sit, it might be hard to believe you'll ever get there. I know it can happen, though. Some of it will come naturally when you begin to feel better about who you are, when you come into your own as a Former Fat Girl. But there are steps you can take to help nudge you into the Uncomfort Zone now, easy things you can do to push yourself to new limits.

The Obstacle: How to Get Over the Fear of the Uncomfortable

Isn't it funny how things can be scary and exciting at the same time? Rickety wooden roller coasters. The King Kong remake. Billy Bob Thornton (well, maybe he's just scary). That's kind of how it is in the Uncomfort Zone. There's got to be a smidgen of fear with every thrill, but taking on something too scary could be counterproductive and drive you right back into the loving arms of Ben & Jerry's. You can ease into the Uncomfort Zone with these fixes.

Former Fat Girl Fixes

Swap stalls.

Every woman I know does it—finds that bathroom stall she can call her own (at work I've got dibs on stall two). Swapping stalls is just a little thing, but even the babiest of baby steps into the Uncomfort Zone can get you used to the idea of making changes, being more flexible, and being out of your routine. Try making a vow to do one little thing differently each week. Instead of going to the same Starbucks every morning, try the one down the block (because unless you live in North Dakota, there's at least one on every block). Or swap your usual latte for a chai. Or grab a takeout dinner for the family and have a picnic at the park—on a weeknight. Mundane? Maybe. Consider this stuff a warm-up for more uncomfortable stuff to come.

Bust a Rut: Five Ways to Make Fitness More Fun and Get More Out of It in the Process

It's a classic fitness conundrum: You work so hard to get into a fitness routine, and once you've achieved that lofty goal, you get bored. And I'm not just talking mentally, either. The fact is, after about six weeks on a particular regimen, your muscles get bored, too. That's why you stop seeing results if you keep doing the same-old-same-old. How can you shake things up? Try these tactics.

1. **Use your mind.** When you're doing a crunch, think about squeezing those stomach muscles first, before you even try to lift your head and shoulders off the ground. Or when you walk, tighten up that butt muscle as you push off. Thinking about the muscle you're trying to work (it's in there, trust me) will make any activity more effective, no learning curve required.

2. **Take the plunge.** It's amazing what those health club programming people come up with: Karaoke spinning, where the instructor moves the mike from bike to bike so the class members can sing along; circus workout, where you take on challenges worthy of high-wire acrobats (don't worry, there is a net); belly dancing, the old Middle Eastern hip-swiveling dance style. All these classes, and more, are available at

clubs around the country. You don't necessarily have to go the weird route; just try something different from what you have been doing. No pressure.

3. **Try a toy.** I'm no gadget-head, but I can appreciate the motivating power of the right piece of gear. A pedometer, for instance, to keep track of your miles can spark a competitive fire in you. The same goes for a heart rate monitor, a gadget that helps you keep tabs on how hard you're working out (or not). Even something as simple as flippers can add a kick to your swimming session.

4. **Tweak your technique.** Picking up your pace for short intervals can make any aerobic activity—walking, running, cycling, elliptical training, and swimming—more interesting and up your calorie burn at the same time. Here is how it works: After warming up for at least three minutes (if you're using a watch), speed up for a minute or two, then drop back down to warm-up pace. Continue alternating faster intervals with slower recovery periods during your workout, ending at a slower pace for three to five minutes. You can time yourself or use landmarks (such as city blocks or streetlights) to mark your intervals.

5. **Change the scenery.** This might mean getting off the treadmill and walking outside or changing your route to a new part of the neighborhood. You might be surprised at how much a simple change of scene can change your attitude about your workout.

Tweak the familiar.

Don't go declaring yourself a vegan if you can't imagine life without cheese, and don't ditch your walking routine in favor of yogarobics (or some equally strange-sounding fitness fusion). Instead, start inching into the Uncomfort Zone with slimmer versions of the foods you know and love and by tweaking (not abandoning) the fitness routine you've worked so hard to establish. Look for lighter versions of your favorite recipes, like I did, or play around in the kitchen yourself (find my tips on page 216). Try a new walking route, add a few hills, or use a toy such as a pedometer to track your miles or a watch to keep time. Give yourself a chance to get used to that uncomfortable feeling instead of shocking your system with things that are completely foreign to you.

Try on your new life: Visit a spa.

I know what you're thinking: *What are you trying to do, torture me? Throw me to the beautiful people so I can relive my years as the designated high school outcast?* Hear me out: Not everyone who goes to spas is chic, fit, and all-around perfect-looking. There are loads of women like you there, particularly at the Former Fat Girl–approved spas I've listed on page 208. Yep, a spa stay is pricey but worth it. Talk about immersing yourself in your new life: Spas are the perfect combination of good, healthy food, fabulous fitness experiences, and ultimate relaxation. A spa is like a controlled environment for a budding Former Fat Girl. It gives you a chance to try on your new life. You can take advantage of all kinds of fitness classes and activities, you get to experience indulgent yet healthy food, and you get a whole lot of TLC, besides. A good spa can show you how pleasurable living the Former Fat Girl life can be. Any trip can be life-changing, but for future Former Fat Girls, a spa stay can be the perfect jump-start. Plus, no one there will know your Fat Girl history.

Don't think about it too much.

If you start focusing on how scary something is, how "not normal" it is, you're going to talk yourself out of it—take, for example, that magazine job I applied for. If I had known that there were 13 million loyal readers with their eyes all over every issue of that magazine, there's no way I would have sent in my resume. What could I possibly write that 13 million people needed to read? That little piece of information would have had the same effect on me as a cold shower on a man in the mood: I would have gone from fired-up to flaccid in a flash.

Let go of the outcome.

I want you to see that you can expect more of yourself than your Fat Girl programming has previously allowed—and succeed. Both parts of that equation are important: As you become more and more confident and more and more comfortable with the feeling of being uncomfortable, you don't want to reach so far out of the range of reality that you start feeling like a failure and wondering why you even tried. The hard thing is knowing what you're really capable of because you've been blinded to some of your own talents for so long. How to deal? Make it your goal to try, simply to act. Measure your success by the chances you take, not by what happens after you take them. Most of us have little control over the outcome of any situation we're in anyway. I had no idea who would be tearing open that envelope containing my resume or how many other applicants were kissing up to him or whether his dog had barfed on his shoes that morning or if he had something against women

Meal Makeovers: How to Slim Down Your Favorite Eats

I may not deserve my own show on the Food Network, but I have learned a thing or two about cooking lighter over the last twenty years. Here are my tips for serving up healthier food for you and your family.

Use low-fat dairy products—not fat-free. There's a reason that the number of completely fat-free products on store shelves has dwindled over the last several years: Many are completely inedible and unsatisfying. But low-fat stuff is a different story. Low-fat cheeses, sour cream, yogurt, and milk are all virtually indistinguishable from the full fat stuff in recipes or alone.

Cut sugar. Reduce the sugar in dessert recipes by one-third, and no one will know the difference. There's a growing low-sugar trend in the grocery store, too. Manufacturers are introducing more and more products with less sugar and no sugar substitutes, such as juices, jams, and jellies. Note: If you want to avoid sugar substitutes, read labels carefully. Sometimes it's hard to tell which products contain them and which ones don't.

Add veggies. Veggies bulk up such dishes as soups and stews without bulking you up in the process. Toss shredded carrots into quick breads, steam extra broccoli and stir it into frozen entrées or meal kits, and top sandwiches with bright greens such as spinach and arugula.

Use whole grains. News flash: Someone took the pastiness out of whole wheat pasta. Whole wheat pasta comes in all shapes and sizes, and is a great way to sneak some fiber into your standard Italian fare. In the bread aisle, make sure the label reads 100% whole grains so that you get all the fiber you're looking for. And for those wheat bread phobes out there (like my husband), check out the new white wheat breads. Your family will never know they're eating the healthy stuff.

Half the sauce. Most sauces are based on butter, oil, or mayo—that's why they taste so good. Instead of trying to choke down a completely naked chicken breast, simply use half the sauce you'd normally serve. The same goes for the meal kits you can find on the shelf at the grocery store: No one says you have to use the entire packet of peanut sauce on your Thai noodles.

Go lean (but not too lean). Choosing leaner cuts in the meat aisle can certainly save you calories and fat, but the very leanest meats are typically too dry and tough to stomach, unless you marinate the heck out of them. For instance, a patty of "extra lean" ground turkey (99 percent fat free) has only 120 calories and 1 gram of fat; the same size patty made of "lean" ground turkey (93 percent fat free) contains 160 calories and 8 grams of fat—but the extra 40 calories and 7 fat grams are worth it. The leaner burger has all the texture of a Birkenstock.

from Texas whose last name began with D. All I could do was make sure I put the right amount of postage on the letter and get it in the mail. That was a victory in itself. You are a winner every time you do something uncomfortable, no matter how it all turns out. Remember that, and it will be easier, I promise, to give fear the boot.

Think: What Would a Former Fat Girl Do?

In those times of doubt when you're afraid to take that risk or go one more step, tap into that Former Fat Girl mind-set by asking yourself, WWFFGD? It's hard to work against that old Fat Girl programming 24-7, but modeling the behavior of your role models can help. It sounds a little goofy, but this tactic helped keep me from bailing when I was going through the three-or-so-month process of getting that senior editor job. Every time I thought, *Who the hell am I to think they'll hire me?* I called on this confident, assertive persona to keep my insecurities from getting the best of me.

I still do, all these years later. This is the way I live my life—try to, anyway: by the secrets in this book. I'm a lifetime member of Weight Watchers, having stayed at a weight of 117 pounds, give or take, for about twenty years now (not counting my pregnant and post-pregnant years). I got that job as a senior editor, moved away from Austin, and hammered out a career in journalism writing about, among other things, health, fitness, and weight loss, helping other women transform their lives the way I did. After a couple of dry runs (one of which lasted about four years), I found a man who loves me (*not* like a buddy), and now I have a son who makes me laugh and runs me ragged every single day. He knows his mommy as someone who stands up for herself, who isn't afraid to make a silly joke, who looks at life as one big, uncomfortable adventure. I wouldn't have any of this—my husband, my son, or my career—if I hadn't made good on that vow I took the day of my ice cream OD so long ago.

And now, Former Fat Girls-to-be, it's your turn to step up. Your future is waiting.

Afterward: What Now?

Once you become a Former Fat Girl, there's one little thing you must do for yourself. You *must* do something to celebrate. Take a trip, go on a shopping spree, hire a skywriter to spread the news. You've done something you never thought you could do, something even the so-called weight loss experts say is impossible. You have pushed and kicked and elbowed your way through all the obstacles. You have carved a new image for yourself, a new body, a new life. You deserve a blowout akin to an Oscar after-party.

Yes, as a newly minted Former Fat Girl, you will have a lot to celebrate—enough to last you a good long while. I, in fact, am still celebrating, and I've been here almost twenty years now. I have never lost sight of how hard it was for me to drop those 70-plus pounds (the size of your average eight-year-old) and how hard it was for me to overcome my fear of reaching for what I wanted—whether it was a guy or a job—and getting hurt in the process. How amazing it is when I can't find a new pair of pants because everything's too big (and not because I wandered into Lane Bryant by mistake) or when I have to struggle over picking one swimsuit out of the five that not only fit but actually look *good*. It's like having to choose one chocolate—*just* one—from a box of Godiva truffles.

I know what you're saying: If those are what you call problems, bring 'em on!

Oh, you will have your share of all the delicious dilemmas you could only dream of having before. And—you knew this was coming—you will face others, too, because being a Former Fat Girl comes with its own set of challenges. You might have an image in your head of the perfect life, the perfect house, the perfect body, the perfect man, all yours when you finally take the weight off. But the reality is a little different, a little less perfect (because you know, reality is *never* perfect). You'll still have your ups and downs; you'll still have to deal with temptations, frustrations, anxiety, even depression. And you won't exactly have food to help you through it, like you did many times before.

The last thing I want to do is put a damper on your celebration, but I do want you to be prepared. You already have some powerful tools to help you deal with anything you'll face in your new life. Wait a minute—you know you can't just drop your INO at the door when you get here, right? You know that continuing to live by the Former Fat Girl secrets is the price of admission, don't you? You know this isn't some diet that just suddenly ends after you've completed your six-week or six-month stretch, yes?

All the things you've learned to get you to this point will

help you rise above the challenges of navigating the world as a Former Fat Girl, but there are particularly difficult issues that I want to make sure you're on the lookout for, issues that I still struggle with even now. Here's one that came up for me just the other day. A woman at work was going from office to office with a bag of Reese's Peanut Butter Cups (the little ones), like a 3:00 P.M. chocolate fairy doling out treats. It was a particularly stressful Monday afternoon. She came to my door, stopped herself, and said, "Oh, I know *you* wouldn't eat one!" No, not me, not *perfect little me*. I was once shamed for eating an entire bag of these things, and now I am shamed because I *won't*?

The interesting thing about this particular woman is that she and I have had this conversation before. She knows I indulge when I want to and that I am a Former Fat Girl, yet she continues to bully. So in this case I said, "Oh, Dolores, I'd *love* one. You know I eat chocolate at least once a day, and these are my favorites." Which is true: I'm especially fond of those little peanut-butter-in-my-chocolate, chocolate-in-my-peanut-butter confections. If it were some crappy knockoff, I wouldn't have bothered. (It's that INO thing; the impostors aren't worth the calories!) But since it was the real deal, I took one and promptly put it in my desk drawer because I'd already had a couple of Hershey's Kisses that afternoon. I would save the Reese's for the next day.

But you see how it happens: The people around you will continue to be hyper-interested in what you eat. They might start thinking of you as some diet freak or some workout freak even when you go to great pains not to appear as though you're forcing your Former Fat Girl ways on them. And then there will be people—some of them men!—lobbing compliments at you, something you may never have experienced before. How do you deal with the wolf whistles? How do you dress this new body of yours? How do you handle life's little (or large) setbacks without fleeing Former Fat Girl world for good? Read on.

The Issue: You Feel Like a Selfish Bitch

Let's start with the hardest one, the one that eats away at your very soul. As a Former Fat Girl you start focusing on getting what you want, on pleasing yourself not just everyone else, remember? But don't be shocked when a little voice in the back of your mind uses the selfish b-phrase. How could you turn down brunch with the girls because of a measly workout? How could you say no to a visit to Mom's and instead go to that movie you've been dying to see? Never mind that you see the girls every week. Never mind that you've always been there when Mom needs you. Your definitions of *selfish* and *bitch* are so completely off, thanks to the Fat Girl programming you're continuing to battle, that anything short of the ultimate sacrifice seems selfish, callous, heartless, and bitchy. You are so used to giving, giving, giving that when you start to take even just a little, that selfish b-phrase comes bubbling up. You may even get it from the people around you who have benefited from your self-sacrificing in the past. But chances are *you* feel it more than anyone else does. Your "selfish bitch" meter is so sensitive that the slightest jolt can set off the alarm.

Mine was particularly difficult to deal with when I went back to work after maternity leave. It was that whole work/life balancing act: I wanted to be with my baby as much as possible while working full-time and trying to get my body back in shape after gaining those forty-two pounds. Early morning and after work exercise were not options, those were precious hours with Johnny that I would never get back. So I decided that I would spend my lunch hours at the gym. I became very protective of that time, but it was difficult for me to deflect lunch invitations without feeling like a selfish bitch. Not to mention the fact that at times I felt that it was politically risky. (I sacrificed a lunchtime workout now and then to satisfy my boss.)

How did I keep from giving in to the little voice that threatened to pull me back into self-sacrificing mode? I tapped into how it felt when my life was all about putting other people first (parents, friends, my boss, my neighbors, anyone who could hold an opinion of me), those days when their happiness was more important than my own. I remembered how empty I felt inside when I was giving everything to everyone else. I remembered the unhealthy resentment I had for the demands and the people pulling on me from every direction. And I remembered that it was my choice whether to give in or not.

The other thing I did, and I continue to do, is surround myself with role models—women like my friend Jill who took a pottery class just for her, who traveled to Italy last year with her sister, who has managed to make monthly girls' night out with her video group for more than ten years, on top of having two kids and a full-time job. I see how her choices feed her soul and how she does it without guilt because she believes she deserves it and is a better mom-wife-sister-friend-employee for it. It helps to have her around when that old people-pleasing programming rears its ugly head.

And then there's always counseling. I have seen a couple of therapists over the last twenty years, especially when I've needed to hear that it's okay to stick up for myself, that saying no, boss, I can't go to lunch with you (but how about a coffee?) doesn't mean I'm a selfish bitch. And what's good about a therapist is that she tells you if you really are a selfish bitch (whereas your mom or a friend might hesitate). You may not like hearing it, but at least you wouldn't be wondering anymore.

The Issue: Your Life Gets Interrupted

Know this: There will be days when you can't stick to your fitness routine and your food plan. You catch a cold; you sprain an ankle; you have an impossible deadline at work; your husband, your child, or your parents get sick. It happens. It's life. Expect it. And in my experience it often happens just when you start feeling good—a little cocky, even. You've finally gotten used to that 6:00 A.M. workout wake-up call, maybe, or you've just gotten the knack of that new kickboxing class, or you've completed your search for lunch takeout that's both healthy and good (no small task).

I have had more life interruptions than I can count, both minor and major. On the more dramatic end, there was the time I wrecked my knee so spectacularly that I ended up going under the knife. It happened one late afternoon when a group of us were out on the lake in Austin, tubing behind a friend's boat. We were sitting on a monster-truck-size inflatable tube that was attached to the boat by a tow rope, apparently to get bumped and battered around as the boat reached top speed. I guess some people think it's fun; if you ask me, it's more like something you'd use to squeeze international secrets out of war prisoners. To make it even worse, the guy driving decided to play a little game with us by zigzagging around the lake in an attempt to dump us into the water. And he started playing in the middle of my turn on the tube. After a few hellish minutes of feeling like a bobblehead, the boat veered left, I swung right, and despite my death grip on the handles, I went flying through the air. Who knew water was so hard when you hit it going eighty miles an hour? I smacked into the surface, my legs at some crazy angle (luckily, I didn't land face-first or I would have ended up looking like I'd stuck my head in a panini press). I knew immediately that something was wrong with my left knee, a hunch that was confirmed when I tried to walk and my leg wouldn't straighten. I borrowed some crutches and limped around for the next couple of days, my knee ballooning up all blue and red. I was too afraid to go to the doctor because I didn't want to hear him say "surgery." I didn't want to hear him say "rest." I didn't want to hear him say "stop." I was scared of the anesthesia, of the pain, of missing too much work. Not only that, after all I had worked for (I was wearing a bikini and looking pretty good when I went slamming into the water), would this stupid tubing incident put me back on the Fat Girl track?

Denial wasn't doing my knee any good; it was clear that I needed professional help. So I went to some orthopedic guy who tried to force my leg out of the 30-degree angle where it was frozen. He's lucky I couldn't get up or I would have punched him. Anyway, it didn't work. Nothing worked. It was either surgery or surgery. So I signed the consent form, slipped into a hospital gown, and prayed I'd end up with a knee that worked a lot better (and hurt a lot less) than the one I had.

The doctor found ligament damage, stitched me up, and sent me on my way in a stupor (this is what they call outpatient surgery). I had to wear a brace to keep my leg completely straight for a couple of days and then spend a few days on crutches. Then, according to the doctor, I could do fifteen minutes a day on the stationary bike. By this time I had worked up to running five miles a day plus playing volleyball and softball once a week. So I was thinking, *"Is he kidding me? Goodbye, size 5 jeans, it's been nice knowin' ya."*

On the verge of giving up or completely freaking out, I dialed frantically back through my Former Fat Girl Fixes for help, and I found it: the whole idea that something is better than nothing. I had a new frame of reference now. I couldn't run—it was physically impossible—but I could get on the bike and see how it feels. I could be faithful to my scaled-down, fifteen-minutes-a-day regimen. I started focusing on what I could do instead of what I couldn't.

And that is what helped me get even stronger and smarter than I was before knee surgery—smarter because I learned that it didn't have to be all or nothing for me. The choice wasn't five miles or five chocolate sundaes. I didn't have to see every setback as a tragedy. There are shades of gray; there are compromises. I just had to be patient, look for them, and give myself time to heal.

Heal I did. I made myself do those fifteen-minute stints—no more, no less—every day. I added more only when my doc told me I could. At the same time I took a hard look at what I was eating, making sure my morning bowl of Bran Chex hadn't inflated, and kept a strict check on my carb-filled friends. That's all I could do, so I did it. I might have gained a few pounds during the six or so months it took me to get back up to speed, but once I (and my fully recovered knee) started hitting the running trails again, I was able to pull out my favorite pair of jeans again.

No matter what kind of interruption you experience, these lessons—being patient with yourself and doing something, however small—can serve you well. When you're keeping vigil at the hospital for a sick parent, you can't exactly stick to your workout schedule, right? But you can and should take any opportunity to move. Walk up the stairs, go out for fresh air, and sneak in a workout when you can—unless, that is, you really need sleep. Because it's all about balance. There's a lot in your life that you can have your way, like your Burger King Whopper (no cheese, no mayo) or the way you start your Saturday morning (with a walk or run, or a coffee and cruller). But when you can't be in the driver's seat, that's when it gets tough. Remember that it's not all or nothing. Remember yourself and your needs even during a crisis (because if you don't choose you at least sometimes, you're not going to be any good to anyone else). Give yourself time to find the shades of gray, to repair and recover. And know that you will bounce back. That's what Former Fat Girls do. It just takes a little while sometimes.

The Issue: You Want to Be the Girlfriend but Don't Know How

This was a tough one for me, even though I became a Former Fat Girl when I was twenty-nine, and two years later I was living with a man who wasn't a blood relative. But it's not like I went from wallflower to ingenue overnight.

I first met Ned after finagling my way into an interview for that senior editor position I eventually landed. It was months after I had sent in my resume with the quirky little poetic cover letter. The poem did its job: I got a call from the managing editor, who asked me to research and write a story about some medical condition so obscure that I can't even remember what it was. If they liked it, I had a good chance of getting hired. I had never really done this sort of research before; most of the stories I'd written were pegged to a certain news event and required maybe one or two interviews. For this one I would have to read up on the problem, find the top sources in the country (much harder than just calling the Chamber of Commerce for a quote), and understand what they were saying well enough to actually write authoritatively about it and in a way other people could understand. At that point in my career, trying to read medical studies and talk to a bunch of doctors and researchers was like asking me to speak Arabic.

But I was all into making myself uncomfortable on this Former Fat Girl adventure, so I dove in, knowing nothing. I spent hours in the library. I yakked it up with all kinds of medical specialists. I discovered *ologies* I never knew existed (you know, otolaryngology, rheumatology, gastroenterology). The story I wrote on my MacPlus with a screen about as big as an iPod Nano was intelligible enough to get me another call from the managing editor—this time a brief phone interview. It was a pretty unmemorable chat. I'm sure we talked about my background, and he asked me how I felt about moving. (The words "I'm there!" might have come out of my mouth.) And then silence.

Two or three weeks went by, and I heard nothing, so I picked up the phone (there's that old "Whatever it takes" from college). I left message after message. No response.

In the meantime, I had planned a trip north to visit my aunt Helen and uncle Bill on Long Island. And then it came to me: The magazine's headquarters were somewhere near Philadelphia. Maybe I could stop over. I mean, everything was all smushed together up there in the Northeast, not like in Texas where you can drive for days before you cross the border.

I put in another call to the magazine, this time to the editor in chief. And he picked up the phone! I croaked out a greeting through my surprise, tried to explain who I was, and said I'd "be in the neighborhood" and would love to come by and meet him. "Set something up with my assistant," he barked, rushing off the phone. And so I did.

After a four-hour drive from Long Island (not exactly in the neighborhood), I landed at the magazine offices in Pennsylvania. During my tour of the joint, I met Ned, who was working in the production department at the time. In case you're imagining one of those MGM moments where eyes meet, music swells, and magic happens, strike that. Not for me. Ned was lanky, about six feet tall, with wavy, light brown hair, deep-set brown puppy dog eyes, and probably the best pair of legs I'd ever seen on a man: long, lean, and muscular. Not that I noticed any of that during the first meeting. The only thing I remembered was that he used a weird expression when he heard where I lived: "Austin? *Sweet*." I'd never heard anyone say that except pro athletes during TV interviews.

By the time I got the job and moved across the country, Ned had taken a job at another magazine at the same company but in a different building. When I saw him again, maybe a full year after I started, he had to remind me that we'd met. That's how clueless I was. Tall, cute Ned made absolutely no first impression on me except for that little bit of jock slang. Where most single women considering moving thousands of miles from home would at the very least be sizing up the dating prospects, I was oblivious. It had still not penetrated my Former Fat Girl mind that, hello—I could actually date this guy.

As I said, I did actually date Ned and did actually live with him (whatever happened to that good girl?), but our relationship was more like a buddies-with-privileges kind of thing.

There was affection, great affection, but no spark, no chemistry like there had been with David. My theory is that I never seriously thought that Ned and I would last. I don't know what it was—maybe his maturity (he was six years younger than me) or maybe his dependency on me (I think he wanted a mommy more than a partner). Maybe it was just the timing of the whole thing. While I had made an uncomfortable choice by becoming physically and intimately involved with Ned—by moving in with him, for God's sake—emotionally I had taken the safe route yet again.

Ned and I lived together for almost four years. One night when we were out to dinner, I said, "We're never going to get married, are we?" It was the first time I'd ever really used the m-word. The next weekend he moved out. A month later he was dating someone else.

Now, talk about your setbacks! I was devastated. Of course I missed him. Of course I mourned. But more than anything, deep down inside I felt like a failure. I knew this thing had gone on too long. I knew nothing would ever come of it. But I wasn't strong enough to end it. I might have been living that uncomfortable life in every other way, but I had gotten cozy and complacent in this relationship.

At least I had started the ball rolling. If I hadn't blurted out what I'd been thinking for, oh, at least two years, who knows how long we would have gone on. So there is that.

This is a bit of a cautionary tale because if there's anything that will be your Achilles' heel, the thing that threatens to hobble you in your new Former Fat Girl life, it's your heart. It's so easy to love the idea of love without seeing the reality of it. It's so easy to love the idea of having a warm body next to you and to forget that maybe you have nothing in common with that particular warm body or that he doesn't treat you like you want him to or that he's not even very nice. He's just there—kind of like the chocolate chip cookies that you continued to nosh on long after you could even taste them anymore just because they were there. Oh, yeah—you've quit that, right? Because it's INO, right? Well, it's INO to stay in a relationship because it's comfortable, too. Just like it's INO to eat a substandard piece of cheap waxy chocolate that won't satisfy your craving anyway, it's INO to give your love life over to a guy who's anything less than top shelf.

The problem is, it's easier to tell the difference between a piece of premium chocolate and the second-rate stuff. It's too bad guys don't come with labels as revealing as the food we buy (Ingredients: saccharine, bullshit, passive-aggressiveness, Rogaine). Part of finally being the girlfriend is being open to being the girlfriend. Try thinking of the guys you meet as potential dates. You don't have to force yourself to be coy, bat your eyelids, or play games. Just think: "Hmmm. Hello, Friday night dinner and a movie." If you doubt the power of your mind to affect the vibe between you, try thinking of the next guy you meet as a potential husband: He will flee, I guarantee.

There are all kinds of books that tell you how to flirt and even classes where you can practice. Partake if you like. But don't think you have to change your personality completely to rev up your dating life. You can telegraph your new openness to girlfriendhood with a few other cues:

- No cussing. Buddies cuss; girlfriends don't.
- Listen. Ask him some wide-open question, like "Why'd you become a tattoo artist?" and let him go. In case you don't already know this, listening is not a common male trait. Show him you are truly a member of the opposite sex by being interested in what he has to say.

- Don't interrupt. Guy-on-guy conversations are all about one-upmanship, so if you have a story to tell or a point to make, wait until he's finished.
- Use your eyes. You've heard it before, I know, but it's a big one for me: Until I look someone in the eye, I feel invisible, like I'm shutting myself off from him. If you look him in the eye, you let him into your world for better or for worse. Take that risk. It's the uncomfortable thing to do.

The eyes, I think, are what made me marry Rick. I was immediately attracted to him, something I had never experienced before (or at least since I first saw Bobby Sherman on that record cover). Rick has these piercing blue eyes that are kind of magnetic; I couldn't help but look into them. With him I never once felt like a buddy. I never wanted to. I am convinced that I was ready as I had never been ready before. If I had met him two, three, or five years before, I wouldn't have even *seen* him. I just wasn't open. I just wasn't ready.

I was thirty-six when I met him, thirty-seven when we started dating, thirty-eight when we married, thirty-nine when I got pregnant, and forty when we had our son, Johnny. So the other thing I would say to you, girls, is "Give yourself time." Anything can happen. Anything is possible—if it's right.

The Issue: You've Got the Body, and Now You Need the Wardrobe

Here in Former Fat Girl World we actually like to shop for clothes—or at least we don't dislike it as much as we used to. Shopping is a whole different game when you don't have to sequester yourself in the plus-size section, isn't it?

One of my big milestones was buying my first pair of size 5 jeans from the juniors' department. For a Former Fat Girl, fitting into a size 5 was the equivalent of a runner breaking the four-minute mile or a scientist winning the Nobel Prize or a Hollywood marriage lasting a year. I remember them distinctly because, frankly, they're still in my closet; I just can't give them up. The brand is Swatch, like the watches. They are regular wash, straight leg, and zip front, and they hit me right at the waist. I bought them at a department store in Houston called Joske's where we always shopped as kids. I wouldn't even have tried them on except that they were on sale and they had somehow gotten mixed in with the size 7's where I was browsing. I held them up to me and they looked big enough, but that didn't mean anything. You know how clothes seem to shrink on the way from the rack to the dressing room.

Anyway, I lugged them in with my other stuff and stepped into them. They made it over my calves. So far so good. They eased over my thighs. Even better. Then I slipped them over my butt. Almost there. Now the true test: the top button. I held my breath and . . . success! Me, the girl who once couldn't wear a size 16 Calvins, had herself a pair of size 5 jeans!

And, boy, did I wear them—for years! I wore them until the hems disintegrated and the bottoms frayed, until the buttonhole threatened to burst and the crotch did, too. I was so proud of them. In high school I had lusted after the button-front Levi's that all the preppy girls wore. I could never figure out how any girl looked good in those things. Even when I was at a reasonable weight, I couldn't manage to find a pair that fit my butt without gaping a good four inches at the waist. These weren't Levi's, but they were the closest thing I could find.

Too bad they were exactly the wrong style for me. It would take years for me to discover this fact, but I had no business wearing high-waisted, straight-leg pants of any kind. High waists—and I'm talking about anything higher than about an inch below your navel—only accentuate any bit of belly you've got. Even if your stomach is as flat as Roseanne Barr's singing voice, high-waisted pants make you look as if you have a gut. No lie. And straight-leg pants? Perfect if I want to look like a tree stump. For little five-foot-four me, flared legs are the thing—not superflared, just slightly flared.

I don't mean to be a self-spoilsport. And I have to say that during that era, the late 80s, there wasn't much of a choice. If you wanted low-rise jeans, you'd have had to get them tailor-made. I tell this story to make a point: Your best wardrobe is one that works with your body, not against it. Some of the rules you've been operating under are probably not going to work with this new body of yours, and I bet they didn't work too well with the old one, either. See, even if you have a few or more extra pounds on you, the high-waist ban applies. No one looks good in high-waisted pants except rail-thin runway models with boy bodies (no waist, no hips). The same goes for pleated pants. That's right: In Former Fat Girl World, pleated pants are verboten.

You are going to have to let go. Let go of the folds of fabric you think are hiding your imperfections. Let go of the idea that the pants fit if you can button them without hyperventilating. Look in the mirror. Are they flattering? If not, they don't fit. Don't buy them. Don't wear them. Go back and find a pair that does.

You can tell I feel strongly about this. I feel strongly about it because I know what a difference it made for me when I discovered, however late in life, that my closet was full of stuff that didn't fit. And I am not talking about pre–Former Fat Girl days. I am talking about size 2 and size 4 clothes that I could and did wear but that didn't do my body justice. You have come too far and worked too hard to let some fashion faux pas undermine you.

Your first task before you hit the mall is to edit your closet. Narrow your collection to the pieces that really work for you. Forget all those reasons for holding on to those short skirts, boxy jackets, and elastic waist pants: *But these were* such *a bargain! Oh, my elderly aunt Minnie gave this to me. I spent a fortune on this dress!* Only pay attention to how each piece fits and flatters. If it doesn't, dump it into the donation box.

This process might sound simple until you try it for yourself. I still struggle with it every time I do a seasonal wardrobe purge. And, hey, I'm not the only one. Putting together a wardrobe of pieces that fit and reflect who you are inside is an issue for women in general. Luckily for those of us who need professional advice, a new book, *Nothing to Wear? A 5-Step Cure for the Common Closet*, can help. The authors, Jesse Garza and Joe Lupo, are the founders of a closet-editing service called Visual Therapy Luxury Lifestyle Consultants. Their book is full of advice on the practical (how to choose pieces that flatter your body type) and the emotional (exercises to help you work through some of those issues that make you cling to clothes that are oh so wrong for you).

It's easier than ever to put these guys' advice into practice without having to spend a fortune on a tailor. The people who make women's clothes have finally figured out that every body is different, and started to offer pieces in multiple cuts and multiple lengths. I'm talking mostly about pants here; they're the hardest thing (next to swimsuits) to buy. Go to Banana Republic, Express, and the Gap, and you will find specific "fits"

Playing Dress-Up

Revise your fashion rules with these Former Fat Girl tips.

Focus on fit, not size.

I know, I know, it's hard to get over your fixation with size, but listen up: I know from experience that you'll look much better in an outfit that fits you than one you've squeezed into because, dammit, you're a size 8! The fact is that there are no size standards in the fashion industry, so Ann Taylor's 8 is probably going to fit differently from Banana's.

Get some flare.

Slightly fuller skirts with a little flare take the emphasis off your hips and help balance out a larger chest. Slightly flared pants worn a little long make short girls look taller, too.

Stay away from bulk.

Pear, apple, persimmon—no matter what your body type, no one looks good in bulky or stiff fabrics. Instead choose clothes with a nice drape, that hug your body (not squeeze it).

Find your waist.

You have one whether you know it or not. A jacket nipped in at the waist shows off your curves; one with a slightly higher waistband can take the emphasis off your tummy.

Go wide.

A wide-leg trouser creates a long, lean line and helps downplay wide hips.

Break right.

A skirt that breaks at the knee can make you look taller and leaner. Note: Miniskirts do not make your legs look longer.

Go with the V.

A v-neck (not too low) actually deemphasizes a large chest.

Stop the sag and bag.

Baggy clothes do not make you look smaller. Trust me. Banish the pleated pants, the tapered legs, the straight-cut jackets, the high-rise pants. Clothes that fit close to your body—not tight, but close—will balance your proportions and allow you to show off your new self without showing too much. And, hey, you deserve to flaunt it a little! You didn't come all this way only to hide your success story under boxy jackets and triple pleats! Allow yourself to shine and say "thank you" when the compliments come!

with specific names in a variety of fabrics. Once you find your fit, shopping is pretty simple. I always know, for instance, that Express's Editor cut will look great on me. (Fitting, isn't it, since I'm an editor?) It probably took my trying on five differ-ent fits in five different sizes to figure that out, but it was worth it. Now I can walk into the store, and the only decision I have to make is whether I want the plaid or the herringbone.

The other basic thing I have learned is that every woman has a waist, and a waist must be accentuated. Whether you're 10, 20, or 50 pounds overweight, what they call a structured jacket will look more flattering than one of those straight jobs. Test the theory for yourself: Try on one structured jacket and one unstructured jacket, and see what you think. I'll bet you'll fall for the fitted version.

The idea of wearing more body-conscious clothing will take some getting used to, I know. It did for me. One way to speed up the process is to watch the amazing transformations on what has become my favorite TV treat: the TLC show *What Not to Wear*. If you haven't seen it, tune in. Two fashion stylists, Stacey London and Clinton Kelly, ambush unsuspect-ing fashion victims, give them specific guidance and a bunch of money, and set them loose in the shopping mecca of New York City. You get to watch as real women learn to find clothes work with their bodies—short, tall, big, small. What's so stunning about these transformations is how choosing one style of jacket over another can completely change your look. You will see right there the magic you can make with the right wardrobe choices. (For a cheat sheet of basic rules for Former Fat Girls, see page 238.)

The next step is to try it for yourself. I suggest starting with a couple of pieces—one jacket and one pair of pants (because who has the dough to replace an entire closetful anyway?). Buy separates so you can wear them with other pieces in your wardrobe. Monitor how you feel when you wear them. Sexier? More confident? Younger? Note whether you get more compliments, even if they're not specifically about what you're wearing. People might notice something different about you, and they might not attribute it to that cute cropped jacket.

The Issue: You Don't Know How to Handle All These Compliments

One of the reasons it's so hard to let go of those baggy, straight-cut duds is the old fear of drawing too much attention to yourself. Hey, I'm the girl who covered her mouth when she smiled, remember? I know what I'm talking about here. It's hard to grasp the fact that you have a body, a womanly body, when your shape starts to emerge from the shadows. Suddenly, there's nowhere to hide: In this body-conscious clothing—the nipped-in waists, the low-rise pants—you feel (as odd as it sounds) naked. You feel exposed.

Some of you will have no problem with the whole attention thing. You might just throw off that beach cover-up and romp around in your tankini without a second thought. You might have no problem basking in the glow of your newfound success, swimming in the sea of compliments coming your way. And, hey, good for you!

I, on the other hand, did everything I could to deflect any compliment I received. I had to make some quip at my own expense ("Oh, I always look good in low light") or find a way to rationalize that it wasn't me who deserved the credit ("Oh, it's these jeans! They suck me in and smooth me out like magic"). I had never been good at taking any kind of compliment, no matter what it was for—a good report card, a decent photo, an insightful answer. But I was particularly bad at fielding flattery based on my appearance.

I have learned, though, to say "thank you." It's amazing how hard it is to squeeze out those two simple words when someone comments on how great your legs look in a skirt. It's amazing how hard it is not to add some kind of explanation to neutralize the whole thing ("It's the boots" or "Thank God for self-tanner!"). I have to force myself to say "thank you" and nothing more, no "But you should see my thighs. Talk about *cellulite.*"

And that's my best advice. *Just say thank you*—even to those unwitting boobs who say stuff like "Oh, my God! You've lost so much weight!" Forgive them; they know not what they say. But they know what they mean. They're trying in their rather clumsy way to tell you how great you look—not to point out how much bigger you once were (even though it might sound like it).

So force yourself to say "thank you" to any and all compliments. It will get easier with practice, I promise. Resist the urge to explain yourself, to rationalize, or to come up with some self-deprecating remark. You might think those quips are funny, but they're really tearing you down little by little. They are denigrating the work you've done; they're pecking away at your well-deserved pride; they're devaluing all the amazing things you've done to get yourself this far.

Inside you may be uneasy with the compliments, with the attention, and with your new self, but in saying "thank you," you're moving in the right direction. Even if you don't quite believe you deserve the props you're getting, the very act of saying "thank you" can help you change all that from the outside in. Every time you say it, you become a little more accepting; you get a little closer to believing you're worthy of having a body you're proud to show off, of living the life you want to live, of being truly and finally happy.

Acknowledgments

If I was really going to thank everyone who made this book possible, I'd have to include the guys who make Hostess Cupcakes, Marshmallow Fluff, and Snickers bars. But I think I'll stick to the people who have encouraged and supported me along the way. My grateful thanks go to:

My agent, Debra Goldstein, and my publisher and editor, Laureen Rowland, who completely got the Former Fat Girl thing from the very beginning and whose feedback helped me push this baby out after a gestation period of, oh, at least eight years.

My friends at *Health* magazine, particularly Doug Crichton, who generously gave me the time to put these words on the page and who has taken many chances on me and my ideas over the years; and Jennifer Deans whose support and friendship have been invaluable.

My enduring friends Jill and Earl and Kim and Mark. I am lucky to have you in my life.

All the friends and colleagues who have been my cheerleaders along the way, especially Pam Fries, Robyn Mait Levine, Eileen Kiernan, Lisa Davis, Abigail Walch, Marty Munson, Anne Krueger, Dimity McDowell.

Barbara Kantrowitz and Kristen Kelch whose offhand comment—"You should write a book"—gave me something to obsess about for years.

My in-laws, Leo and Christine Horton, who have dropped everything to come to our rescue too many times to count.

My parents, Joseph and Barbara Delaney, and my brothers and sister who loved me through thick and thin (ha!), even when I didn't feel like there was much reason to. You created a stable jumping-off place that was there for me when I finally had the courage to make the leap.

My husband, Rick Horton, and our son, Johnny. You keep me laughing, singing, dancing, and grounded in the things that matter most.

About the Author

isa Delaney, an award-winning magazine writer and editor, is currently special projects director at *Health* magazine. She has spent the majority of her journalism career covering diet, fitness, nutrition, and health for women's consumer magazines and has written for *Prevention, Vogue, Men's Health, Cooking Light,* and *Reader's Digest.* Since becoming a Former Fat Girl, Lisa has married the man she loves, moved to Birmingham, Alabama, and now wears a size 2.